THE CLINICAL CONVERSATIONALIST

"The greatest compliment that was ever paid me
was when one asked me what I thought, and attended to my answer."
—*Henry David Thoreau*

THE CLINICAL CONVERSATIONALIST

A Patient Educator's Guide to Working With Insomnia Clients

LINDA ROSENBERY

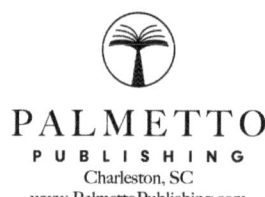

PALMETTO
PUBLISHING
Charleston, SC
www.PalmettoPublishing.com

Copyright © 2023 by Linda Rosenbery

All rights reserved

No portion of this book may be reproduced, stored in a retrieval system, or transmitted in any form by any means–electronic, mechanical, photocopy, recording, or other–except for brief quotations in printed reviews, without prior permission of the author.

Paperback ISBN: 979-8-8229-3304-0
eBook ISBN: 979-8-8229-3305-7

To Dr. Linda Harper,

Your dedicated career in exploring the quantum physics of the human mind, especially in the entanglements of helping with a big heart, has profoundly inspired me. Your influence is a thread that runs through this book, reminding us of the importance of nurturing our compassion while serving others.

Dr. Harper is author of the following books:
Give to Your Heart's Content: Without Giving Yourself Away
The Power of Joy in Giving to Animals
The Tao of Eating: Feeding Your Soul Through Everyday Experiences with Food
Eat! Rediscover Your Best Natural Relationship with Food
Give: A Guide to Discovering the Joy of Everyday Giving

Table of Contents

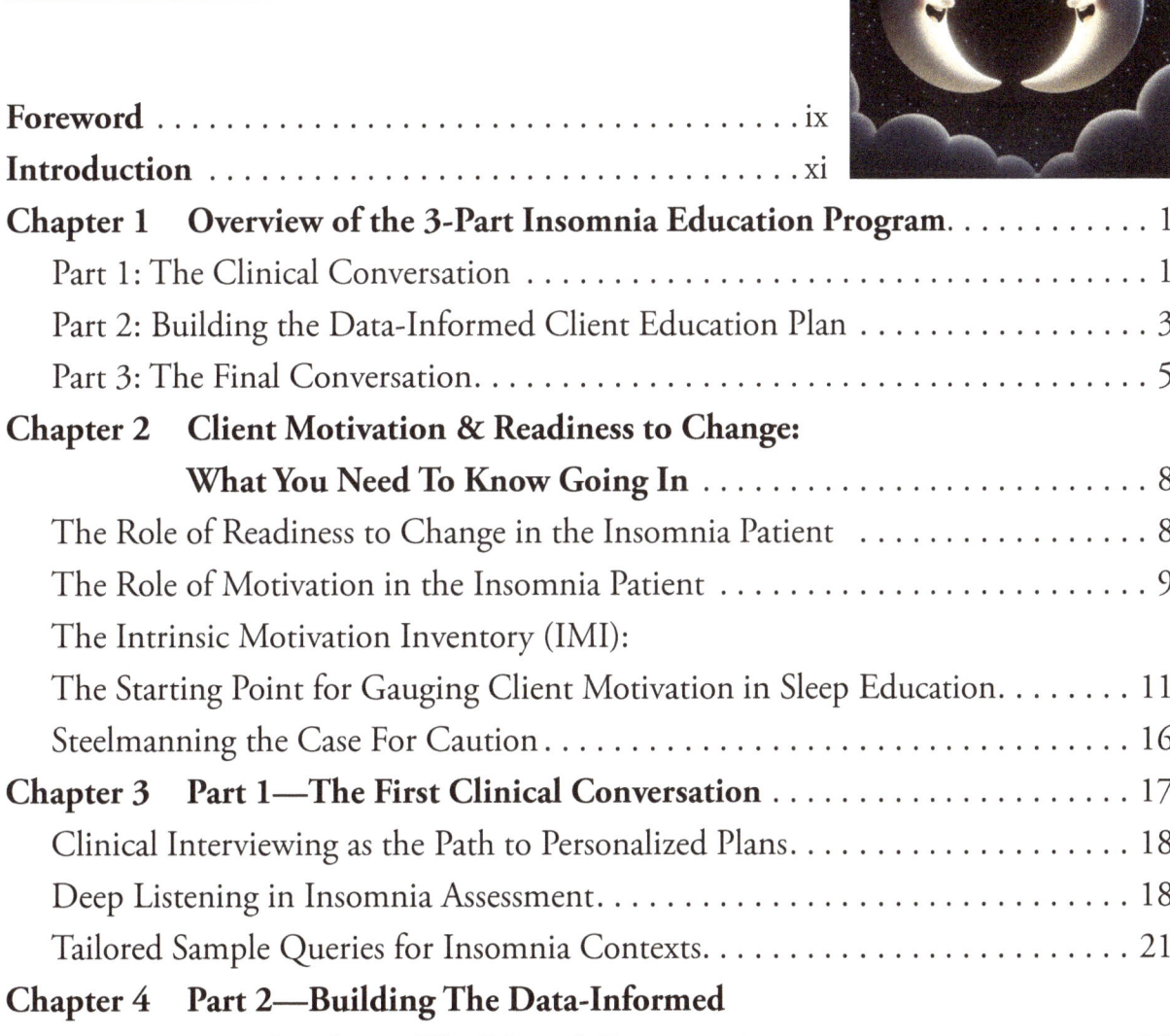

Foreword ix
Introduction xi
Chapter 1   Overview of the 3-Part Insomnia Education Program. 1
  Part 1: The Clinical Conversation 1
  Part 2: Building the Data-Informed Client Education Plan 3
  Part 3: The Final Conversation. 5
**Chapter 2   Client Motivation & Readiness to Change:
         What You Need To Know Going In** 8
  The Role of Readiness to Change in the Insomnia Patient 8
  The Role of Motivation in the Insomnia Patient 9
  The Intrinsic Motivation Inventory (IMI):
  The Starting Point for Gauging Client Motivation in Sleep Education. 11
  Steelmanning the Case For Caution 16
Chapter 3   Part 1—The First Clinical Conversation 17
  Clinical Interviewing as the Path to Personalized Plans. 18
  Deep Listening in Insomnia Assessment. 18
  Tailored Sample Queries for Insomnia Contexts. 21
**Chapter 4   Part 2—Building The Data-Informed
         Data Synthesis: The Mental Computation**. 25
  How the Insomnia Motivation Inventory (IMI)
  Affects Which Remedies to Suggest 26
  First Look at What's Trending in Insomnia Remedies 27
  Creative Presentation of the Education Plan. 29

vii

Chapter 5   Part 3—The Final Clinical Conversation............................ 32
   Presenting the Tailored Plan... 32
   Wrapping Up the Session: Empowering the Client for Immediate
   Implementation.. 34
   When Your Client Does Not Want to Say Goodbye........................ 37
   "One More Thing Before You Go"—
   Give Your Clients A Heads Up On Cognitive Distortions................. 38
      Insomnia with Shiftwork.. 40
      Insomnia with PTSD... 42
      Insomnia with Anxiety... 44
      Insomnia with Depression... 45
      Insomnia with Obstructive Sleep Apnea............................... 47
      Insomnia with Bipolarity... 49
      Insomnia with Medication-Induced Insomnia........................ 50

Chapter 6   The Spectrum of Modern Insomnia Remedies........................ 53
   Insomnia Remedies Alphabetized... 53

Chapter 7   Insomnia: Five Case Studies.. 61
   The Tired Teacher.. 63
   Night Owl Anthony... 73
   The Nocturnal Art Student.. 81
   The Restless Retiree.. 91
   Joe, The Sleep-Seeking Soldier..102

Epilogue: The Illusion of Sleep Health:
When Good Enough Sleep is Good Enough..................................113
References..121

Foreword

The critical impact of insomnia on overall health and quality of life cannot be overstated. As a sleep physician, I have seen firsthand how this condition can be both a harbinger and a concomitant of various medical and psychological disturbances. It is imperative that insomnia is addressed with urgency. Prompt intervention may avert the entrenchment of chronic sleep difficulties and stave off associated risks like depression, anxiety, and cardiovascular disease.

The management of insomnia demands not only an immediate response but consistent follow-up. It is essential for clients to receive timely assessments and for their progress to be meticulously monitored. This proactive surveillance ensures that treatment plans remain dynamic, evolving responsively to the client's journey and needs.

Central to this approach is the recognition of each client's unique narrative of insomnia. Influenced by an array of factors, from lifestyle to stress levels and underlying health conditions, the complexity of their experiences defies a standardized fix. The onus is on us, the sleep physicians, to curate treatment strategies that are as individualized as the clients we serve, thereby reinforcing their autonomy and active participation in the healing process.

Paradoxical insomnia, characterized by a stark divergence between a client's subjective experience of sleep and objective findings, presents a compelling challenge to the field of sleep medicine. It underscores the imperative for a unified standard in defining and quantifying sleep state misperception. My perspective as a sleep physician positions insomnia primarily as a symptom interwoven with other medical or psychological conditions, rather than as an isolated disorder. This view is subject to discourse within the sleep medicine community, reflecting a spectrum of interpretations and theories. Yet, I acknowledge the dialectical essence of this debate, recognizing the value of diverse perspectives in enriching our understanding and treatment of insomnia.

In the context of these reflections, Linda Rosenbery's curriculum emerges as a significant tool to work with insomnia clients. In its pages, Rosenbery elucidates a three-part program that champions the necessity of individualized client education. Her emphasis on dialogue as a tool for therapeutic engagement and her insightful case studies provide an invaluable resource for both practitioners and clients alike. This guide aligns seamlessly with the principles I uphold in my practice—affirming the indispensability of personalized care in the pursuit of sleep health and well-being.

Jonathan Warren, MD, ABSM
Itasca, Il
November 2023

Introduction

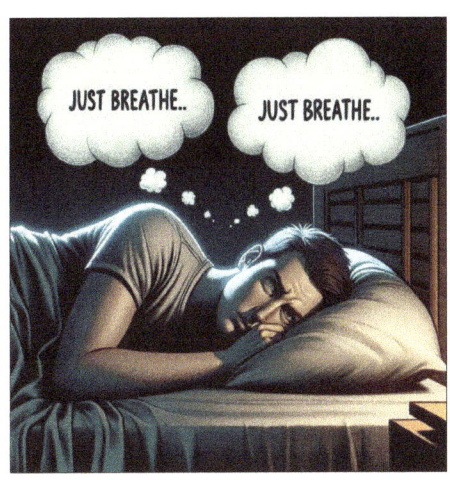

"I suffer from insomnia, and I swear, if someone tells me one more time to 'just breathe' I am going to snap."

This quote captures the frustration many insomnia sufferers feel when faced with generic solutions, doesn't it? It underscores the need for a more nuanced, individualized approach rather than a standardized fix.

There is a huge shortage of us—trained, compassionate humans to work with insomnia sufferers. This pressing need is underscored by insights from the Insomnia Daytime Symptoms and Impacts Questionnaire (IDSIQ) and Grandner et al.'s (2023) seminal study. Their research, examining the impact of untreated insomnia on one million adults, reveals profound daytime effects like increased fatigue, dizziness, and cognitive impairments, and links untreated insomnia to serious health issues, including hypertension, psychiatric disorders, and metabolic disturbances. These findings highlight the critical necessity for healthcare professionals to promptly address insomnia, advocating for interventions that improve both nighttime sleep and daytime functioning.

You might find the insomnia remedies listed in chapter six too generic or simple, something one could easily Google. And you would have a valid point. Playing devil's advocate, what would you do if I told you that nothing works to remedy insomnia? Like the Joe Cocker lyric: "Would you get up and walk out on me?"

You will hear this over and over from patients: "I've tried it all, and nothing works for me." Insomnia clients will be tough on you and this is when you will need to consider a conceptual rethink of insomnia education. Despite the availability of insomnia remedies online, the role of the patient educator is to help clients navigate this sea of good information, debunk the bad, and provide a caring, listening ear. Often, after you let a client voice their frustration, their emotional temperature stabilizes to a point where they are able to revisit some of the same recommendations.

What sets our approach apart is the integration of these remedies with a coaching perspective. Think of it this way: Many dive into gym memberships and expensive workout gear with gusto, only to find that their most strenuous exercise is lifting their credit card to pay for it all. Similarly, the simplest interventions, though seemingly straightforward, greatly benefit from support.

Your expertise lies in shaping insomnia strategies into something more potent—a distinct and deliberate, individualized plan that tackles human inertia, gets the client to own the plan, igniting a spark of change, motivating them to embark on their journey to better sleep from the moment they leave your conversation.

In my 20 years of counseling clients, primarily those with substance misuse, insomnia has been a significant hurdle in the early days of abstinence. This experience has deeply informed my approach and understanding of the complexities of insomnia. As a Patient Educator or Counselor, you will embark on this transformative sleep journey together with your client. Your client's good night's sleep is not just a dream; it's a conversation away.

Acknowledging the Pillars of Insomnia Expertise

Gratitude to the American Academy of Sleep Medicine

Just a brief 20-minute drive from my office lies the esteemed American Academy of Sleep Medicine (AASM), an institution I have come to deeply admire and respect. Over the years, attending their annual conferences in all parts of the U.S. has not only broadened my horizons but also deepened my appreciation for the psychology of sleep medicine. Each session I have attended, especially those focusing on the psychology of sleep, has been poignant and directly relevant to my practice.

Standing on the Shoulders of Giants

I would be remiss not to acknowledge the pivotal role of leaders in behavioral health within Sleep Medicine. Institutions like the Centers for Sleep Research at renowned establishments—the Cleveland Clinic, University of Pittsburgh, and Stanford University—have been instrumental in advancing our collective understanding.

While this guide does not delve into the licensed realm of CBT-I techniques, it is noteworthy that the resonance of cognitive restructuring approaches championed by patient educators is ubiquitous in self-help paradigms worldwide. It is this universality that underscores the profound potential and relevance of the 'Clinical Conversationalist' approach.

CHAPTER 1

Overview of the 3-Part Insomnia Education Program

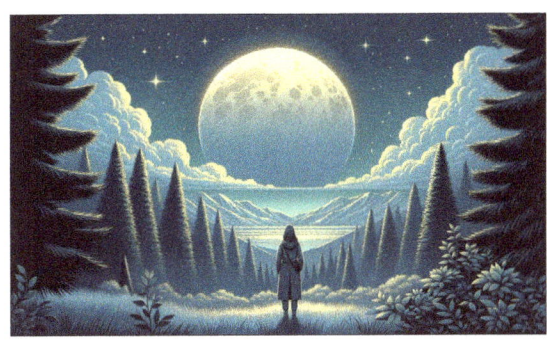

Part 1: The Clinical Conversation

Foundations of the Program

The Clinical Conversation is a crucial phase in the 3-Part Insomnia Education Program. It is rooted in the principles of ethical client education and prioritizes mutual understanding and compassion. This initial phase is not merely about gathering information; it's a process of building a trusting relationship where clients feel valued, heard, and understood. The approach is deeply influenced by Carl Rogers' client-centered therapy, focusing on active listening and empathetic engagement.

Defining the Clinical Conversationalist

The role of a "Clinical Conversationalist" is central to this phase, representing a unique blend of deep knowledge and the art of conversation. This term symbolizes the union of precise educational expertise and the soft skills necessary for meaningful interaction with patients. An effective educator in this context is not just an expert on insomnia but excels in creating a bridge between complex clinical knowledge and the patient's personal experience.

The Art of Clinical Interviewing

Educators in this program are skilled conversationalists, adept at creating an environment of unconditional positive regard. This approach goes beyond merely asking questions; it involves crafting a space where clients feel safe to share their experiences and struggles with insomnia. Active listening is emphasized, allowing clients to guide the conversation, revealing their unique challenges and perspectives on insomnia.

Example: A client discusses how their insomnia has evolved beyond being just stress-related. The educator's subtle response, acknowledging this evolution, exemplifies the depth of understanding and empathetic engagement.

Deep Listening and Shaped Responses

Deep listening, akin to the 'longform' approach used in podcasting, is a key technique employed in this phase. Educators allow clients to steer the conversation, ensuring a comprehensive understanding of the client's insomnia. This stage involves preparing for interviews, setting an atmosphere conducive to open conversation, and employing strategies like paraphrasing and reflective responses to make the client feel respected and understood.

The Power of Conversation in Therapy

The act of conversing about insomnia is an integral part of the therapeutic process. When individuals articulate their experiences, it serves multiple transformative purposes:

1. **Validation and Normalization**: Discussing insomnia helps individuals understand they are not alone, providing solace through empathy and shared experiences.
2. **Self-awareness and Insight**: Speaking about their challenges allows patients to gain deeper insights into their sleep patterns, triggers, and behaviors, aiding in the identification of effective therapeutic strategies.
3. **Therapeutic Alliance**: The rapport and trust built with the patient educator become the foundation for effective treatment, like Cognitive Behavioral Therapy for Insomnia (CBT-I).

Traits of an Exceptional Conversationalist

An effective Clinical Conversationalist embodies several key traits:

1. **Active Listening**: Giving full attention, making the speaker feel heard and understood.

2. **Empathy**: Understanding and sharing the feelings of others.
3. **Open-mindedness**: Being receptive to new ideas and discussing a variety of topics without bias.
4. **Clarity**: Articulating thoughts and ideas clearly, especially when dealing with complex subjects.
5. **Adaptability**: Adjusting the conversation's tone, pace, and content to suit the listener's needs.
6. **Curiosity**: Asking open-ended questions and showing genuine interest in the responses.
7. **Respect**: Maintaining respectfulness even during disagreements, avoiding dominating the conversation.

Part 2: Building the Data-Informed Client Education Plan

Synthesizing Client Information

The second part of the program focuses on developing a data-informed client education plan, synthesizing information from clinical conversations. Patient educators perform a type of mental computation, integrating each piece of shared information as a critical data point. This involves strategic note-taking and the creation of visual flowcharts, aiding in this complex task of aligning clients' unique circumstances with the most suitable interventions.

The Role of the Insomnia Motivation Inventory (IMI)

An essential element in this process is the Insomnia Motivation Inventory (IMI). This tool assesses a client's readiness to engage with different insomnia remedies. High IMI scores in areas like Interest/Enjoyment suggest a client's inclination towards more complex remedies, such as Clinical and Therapeutic Methods. In contrast, lower scores in domains like Effort may indicate a preference for solutions like Natural Aids and Supplements or Environmental Adjustments, requiring less initial and ongoing input.

Example: A client's high IMI scores in Perceived Competence could lead to the recommendation of Traditional Eastern Remedies, requiring sustained effort and engagement, whereas another client with lower scores in Effort might start with simpler solutions like Environmental Adjustments.

Trending Insomnia Remedies and Customization

Educators stay updated with trending insomnia remedies, ensuring the education plan incorporates the most effective strategies. The remedies are arranged in a hierarchy based on the commitment they typically require, from the most to the least demanding, and are adapted to each client's unique situation and motivational readiness.

Creative Presentation of the Education Plan

Designing the Paper Plan

When constructing the paper plan, marrying aesthetic appeal with practical functionality is key. The plan should be visually engaging and organized to facilitate understanding and retention. It should cater to individual learning styles, incorporating diagrams or flowcharts for visual learners and succinct summaries for those who prefer text.

Crafting an Engaging PowerPoint

An effective PowerPoint presentation for client education involves more than static slides and bullet points. It should integrate elements like relevant storytelling, client-centered scenarios, and interactive questions. Slide transitions and animations, short video clips, and sound bites can be used to foster a dynamic learning environment.

Utilizing Visual Aids

Visual aids are instrumental in making the education plan more accessible. Charts, models, and infographics can serve as focal points for discussion and act as mnemonic devices. The use of color coding within the plan serves as both a visually stimulating experience and an organizational tool, aiding in memory retention.

Embracing Digital Adaptations

Digital literacy's rise necessitates the adaptation of these mediums for digital consumption. Digital documents can be rich with hyperlinks for an exploratory approach, and PowerPoint presentations can include live polls and interactive elements for real-time engagement. Interactive infographics and clickable charts in the digital realm provide clients with autonomy to navigate their educational journey.

Building the Data-Informed Client Education Plan is a critical phase of the 3-Part Insomnia Education Program, where patient educators transform the insights gathered from clinical conversations into actionable strategies for insomnia management. By using tools like the IMI and incorporating the latest trends in insomnia remedies, educators are able to construct customized, effective, and engaging education plans that resonate with each client's unique needs and preferences. This process exemplifies the program's commitment to providing personalized, empathetic, and informed care to individuals struggling with insomnia.

Part 3: The Final Conversation

Finalizing and Implementing the Plan

The final phase, "The Final Conversation," is a critical juncture where the tailored education plan is presented and refined collaboratively with the client. This phase ensures complete understanding and confidence in the plan's execution. It's a crucial session, possibly the last formal meeting, where the client must leave feeling empowered and capable of managing their insomnia.

Example: The educator might start with "Here's your personalized sleep plan. Let's go through this together," encouraging the client to actively participate and mark areas in the plan that resonate or need clarification.

Addressing Cognitive Distortions

A significant aspect of this final phase is addressing cognitive distortions. Educators work with clients to identify and challenge negative self-talk. Techniques such as cognitive restructuring are employed to replace irrational thoughts with more balanced perspectives. This part of the session can be crucial for breaking barriers to effective insomnia management.

Example: For a client with anxiety-related insomnia, the educator might challenge the belief "If I don't sleep well tonight, everything will go wrong tomorrow" with a more rational thought like "One restless night doesn't determine my entire day".

Empowering the Client for Immediate Implementation

This section focuses on concluding the session on a motivational note, equipping the client with practical steps for immediate action. Emphasizing the importance of a positive mindset and starting with small, manageable changes can set the stage for immediate and long-term success.

Example: An educator might suggest, "Tonight let's start with something simple, like finding a soothing podcast to listen to as you wind down," helping the client visualize the first step they can take that very night.

Scheduling Follow-up and Ongoing Support

Discussing ongoing support is vital as this might be the last scheduled session. Emphasizing the importance of tweaking the plan and utilizing support networks is key. The availability of various resources, such as online forums and support groups, is outlined to provide continued guidance.

Example: The educator might offer to schedule a follow-up session or check in after a week, reinforcing the message that the client's journey towards better sleep health is ongoing and supported.

When Your Client Does Not Want to Say Goodbye

In cases where clients express a desire to continue sessions, educators are advised on how to handle such situations. Discussions about extended sessions, alternative payment options, and transparent communication about the organization's policies are encouraged to ensure clients feel supported in their journey.

Comprehensive Cognitive Distortion Education

The program includes a detailed exploration of cognitive distortions across various insomnia contexts, such as shift work, Post Traumatic Stress Disorder (PTSD), anxiety, depression, obstructive sleep apnea, bipolarity, and medication-induced insomnia. By recognizing and addressing these distortions through cognitive-behavioral therapy and other interventions, clients can significantly improve their sleep and overall mental well-being.

The 3-Part Insomnia Education Program, with its final phase focusing on collaborative plan finalization, cognitive distortion management, and continued support, offers a comprehensive solution for individuals struggling with insomnia. It underscores the program's commitment to providing a holistic, personalized approach to sleep health, ensuring clients are equipped with the knowledge, strategies, and support needed for effective insomnia management.

CHAPTER 2

Client Motivation & Readiness to Change: What You Need To Know Going In

The Role of Readiness to Change in the Insomnia Patient

There is an undeniable truth in working with insomnia clients: their readiness for change and motivation are dynamic elements, entirely beyond the control of anyone but the client themselves. This realization is key, as it relinquishes control, grounding our approach in realistic expectations and fostering a necessary flexibility throughout the therapeutic journey. This perspective is especially crucial when applying the Transtheoretical Model of Behavior Change, a framework developed by James Prochaska and Carlo DiClemente. This model, with its six distinct stages, offers a deep insight into the varying readiness levels of clients, highlighting the importance of individualized and adaptive strategies in managing sleep health:

1. **Precontemplation**: In this initial stage, insomnia clients may not recognize the need to change their sleep habits. For instance, a client might consistently underestimate the benefits of regular sleep patterns and overemphasize the challenges in changing their night routines.
2. **Contemplation**: At this point, clients start acknowledging the need for better sleep hygiene. However, ambivalence may still be present, as seen in clients who understand the importance of good sleep but struggle with the idea of changing their long-standing habits.
3. **Preparation**: Clients now begin to take small but significant steps towards change, often informed by online research. This could include setting a consistent bedtime or reducing screen time before sleep, marking the start of tangible planning and initial behavior adjustments.

4. **Action**: Here, clients actively engage in modifying their behaviors to improve sleep quality. This stage demands a substantial commitment and often involves major lifestyle adjustments like adhering to a strict sleep schedule or engaging in deliberate routines before bed. It's common for clients to seek help from a sleep physician and work closely with a sleep educator during this phase.
5. **Maintenance**: After achieving behavior change, the focus shifts to sustaining these new habits and preventing relapse. This can be challenging, as clients must continually reinforce their new sleep patterns to make them a permanent part of their lifestyle.
6. **Termination or Relapse**: In some interpretations of the model, this final stage is reached when clients no longer feel at risk of reverting to old habits and are confident in their new, healthier sleep patterns. However, a return to old habits and not following their education plan could lead them back to the pre-contemplation stage.

It's important to note that these stages are not strictly linear. Clients may oscillate between stages, and relapse is considered a normal part of the change process. This non-linear progression underscores the model's emphasis on personal and gradual change, moving away from a standardized fix approach.

By recognizing where a client is in these stages, you can tailor your educational and therapeutic approaches to their specific readiness level, thus enhancing the effectiveness of your interventions in promoting long-term sleep health.

The Role of Motivation in the Insomnia Patient

The evolution of sleep medicine has mirrored broader shifts in healthcare, moving from a predominantly pharmacological orientation to an increasingly multifaceted, client-centered approach. While medication undoubtedly retains its role, especially in acute cases, the spotlight has increasingly fallen on the interplay of psychological, behavioral, and educational factors. Specifically, the concept of learner motivation has come to occupy a key position in this expanded therapeutic landscape. Understanding how these variables coalesce allows healthcare providers, including physicians and client educators, to design more effective and personalized treatment strategies.

The case studies in Chapter 7 exemplify this concept vividly. For instance, Janice, the Tired Teacher, battles cognitive hyperarousal, a common trigger of insomnia. Her case emphasizes the need for interventions that focus on cognitive behavioral techniques to manage her nighttime thoughts, enhancing her motivation for treatment engagement. Similarly, Anthony, a night-shift security guard, confronts lifestyle and environmental factors that disrupt his sleep. His case underscores the necessity for strategies that address both circadian rhythm disturbances and emotional well-being.

Both emotional and cognitive variables significantly affect a client's willingness to engage in recommendations for change. For clients like Janice and Anthony, understanding their emotional triggers and cognitive roadblocks can elevate the their motivation to fully engage with their treatment.

Self-Determination Theory (SDT) lays the foundation for fostering intrinsic motivation by meeting the psychological needs of autonomy, competence, and relatedness. For insomnia clients, this translates into having more control over their treatment decisions, a better understanding of their condition, and a supportive relationship with healthcare providers. Addressing these needs not only boosts engagement but also helps internalize behavioral changes for long-term improvement.

Hands-On Techniques for elevating motivation, such as motivational interviewing, trust-building, and feedback mechanisms, are illustrated in the case studies. Applying these techniques can help clinicians break down psychological barriers that impede treatment adherence in insomnia clients. Trust and open dialogue can substantially elevate motivation, making clients more receptive to treatment.

Self-Efficacy, or the belief in one's capability, is crucial in the successful tapering of medication for insomnia clients. By nurturing a belief in their ability to manage their condition, clients are more likely to be actively involved in their treatment, further enhancing their intrinsic motivation.

The construct of motivation in the insomnia client is far from monolithic; there are shades of color from various theories, emotional and cognitive elements, hands-on techniques, and educational practices, a palette of factors that, when appropriately addressed, can profoundly influence the success of insomnia education plans. Specifically, they underscore the importance of involving client educators alongside physicians to deepen client understanding and facilitate long-term behavioral change.

The Intrinsic Motivation Inventory (IMI): The Starting Point for Gauging Client Motivation in Sleep Education

The Intrinsic Motivation Inventory (IMI):
A Preliminary Tool for Client Motivation Assessment in Sleep Education

In the realm of sleep education, assessing a client's intrinsic motivation is a continued effort to gain insight to tailor an effective education plan. The Intrinsic Motivation Inventory (IMI) serves as an essential preliminary tool in this process. It can be effectively administered by a sleep physician or a referral source prior to initiating the education program. This multidimensional tool is designed to evaluate various aspects of a client's motivation, encompassing Interest/Enjoyment, Perceived Competence, Effort, and other key dimensions.

Validated across diverse settings, the IMI provides a nuanced understanding of each client's motivational landscape, laying the groundwork for a customized and impactful sleep education journey. By integrating the IMI early on, sleep educators can glean valuable insights, enabling them to align their educational strategies with the unique motivational profiles of their clients.

The IMI comes in multiple versions with varying numbers of items and subscales, allowing educators to choose what best suits their specific research questions or client needs. Here are the core subscales of the IMI and their relevance in insomnia.

IMI Core Subscales
1. Interest/Enjoyment: The cornerstone of intrinsic motivation, this subscale helps educators gauge how engaged clients are in the education process, making it easier to adapt materials or strategies to sustain interest.
2. Perceived Competence: By assessing how capable clients feel in managing their sleep issues, educators can fine-tune the complexities of the interventions they offer.
3. Effort: This subscale enables educators to understand the extent to which clients are willing to put in the work, be it in maintaining sleep logs or following through on relaxation techniques.
4. Value/Usefulness: Understanding the client's perception of the utility of the sleep education process allows for more targeted conversations around the long-term benefits of behavioral changes.
5. Felt Pressure and Tension: A negative predictor of intrinsic motivation, this subscale can signal when a client might be feeling overwhelmed, allowing for timely adjustments in the education plan.
6. Perceived Choice: Enhancing this facet can elevate the client's sense of autonomy, encouraging active participation in the selection of insomnia remedies or other treatment options.
7. Relatedness: Though still under validation, this new addition could help educators gauge the quality of their therapeutic alliance with the client.

When you look at the scores from this motivation scale, think about the needs and goals of your patients. Higher scores in the enjoyment section, for example, mean the patient finds the treatment activities enjoyable, which is a good sign. Unlike some complicated tools, this scale doesn't set strict 'high' or 'low' score limits. Rather, you'll want to use the scores to track how a patient's motivation changes over time or to compare between patients.

With this scale, you have the flexibility to zoom in on the aspects most important for your insomnia education program. This user-friendly tool helps ensure you understand the motivational factors at play, which is crucial for creating effective and personalized education plans for your patients.

Sample IMI Survey

IMI Survey Instructions

Thank you for participating in our Insomnia Education Program. Before we begin, we'd like to understand how you're feeling about the upcoming activities. Your honest feedback is crucial for tailoring the program to better meet your needs. Please know that whether you're excited, indifferent, or even reluctant, your feelings will not affect the quality of care and guidance you'll receive throughout this program. Honesty is key. Please take a few moments to circle the number that best reflects your agreement with each statement.

Interest/Enjoyment

Scoring Scale:
- 1: Not at all true
- 2: Mostly not true
- 3: Somewhat not true
- 4: Neither true nor untrue
- 5: Somewhat true
- 6: Mostly true
- 7: Very true

1. I am looking forward to the activities in this program.
   1 2 3 4 5 6 7
2. I think the upcoming program will be fun.
   1 2 3 4 5 6 7
3. I expect the activities in this program to be interesting.
   1 2 3 4 5 6 7

4. I think this program will be enjoyable.
   1 2 3 4 5 6 7
5. As I prepare for this program, I'm thinking about how much I'll enjoy it.
   1 2 3 4 5 6 7

Perceived Competence

Scoring Scale:
- 1: Not at all true
- 2: Mostly not true
- 3: Somewhat not true
- 4: Neither true nor untrue
- 5: Somewhat true
- 6: Mostly true
- 7: Very true

1. I believe I will be good at the activities in this program.
   1 2 3 4 5 6 7
2. Compared to others who have taken this program, I think I will do well.
   1 2 3 4 5 6 7
3. I expect to feel competent after completing this program.
   1 2 3 4 5 6 7
4. I believe I will be satisfied with my performance in this program.
   1 2 3 4 5 6 7

Effort/Importance

Scoring Scale:
- 1: Not at all true
- 2: Mostly not true
- 3: Somewhat not true

- 4: Neither true nor untrue
- 5: Somewhat true
- 6: Mostly true
- 7: Very true

1. I plan to put a lot of effort into this program.
   1 2 3 4 5 6 7
2. I will try my best during this program.
   1 2 3 4 5 6 7
3. Doing well in this program is important to me.
   1 2 3 4 5 6 7

Value/Usefulness

Scoring Scale:
- 1: Not at all true
- 2: Mostly not true
- 3: Somewhat not true
- 4: Neither true nor untrue
- 5: Somewhat true
- 6: Mostly true
- 7: Very true

1. I believe participating in this program could be valuable to me.
   1 2 3 4 5 6 7
2. I think that participating in this program will be useful for improving my sleep.
   1 2 3 4 5 6 7
3. I am willing to participate in this program again as it has value for my well-being.
   1 2 3 4 5 6 7

4. I believe that this program could help me with my insomnia.
   1 2 3 4 5 6 7
5. I consider this program to be an important step for my health.
   1 2 3 4 5 6 7

Thank you for taking the time to complete this survey. Your feedback will help us make this program as beneficial as possible for you.

Steelmanning the Case For Caution

Dr. Linda Harper, an esteemed clinical psychologist with expertise in the fluid nature of client motivation in clinical settings, offers a thoughtful critique on the use of motivational questionnaires. Her skepticism is grounded in the complexity of human psychology and the limitations inherent in self-reported data.

Dr. Harper emphasizes that responses to these questionnaires may not purely reflect motivation but often capture a mix of other psychological states, such as defiance, frustration, or a defensive mindset. This conflation can lead to misleading interpretations of a client's true motivational levels. She also points out the variability and context-sensitivity of human emotions and motivations. These can fluctuate with changing circumstances, making the reliability of such tools in capturing a consistent measure of motivation questionable.

Additionally, Harper notes the paradox of clients with low motivation scores often excelling in therapy, and clients with high motivation scores facing disillusionment when high expectations are unmet, potentially overshadowing genuine progress. Dr. Harper's perspective calls for a cautious approach to motivational questionnaires in therapy, advocating for a more holistic evaluation of clients' therapeutic journeys.

CHAPTER 3

Part 1–The First Clinical Conversation

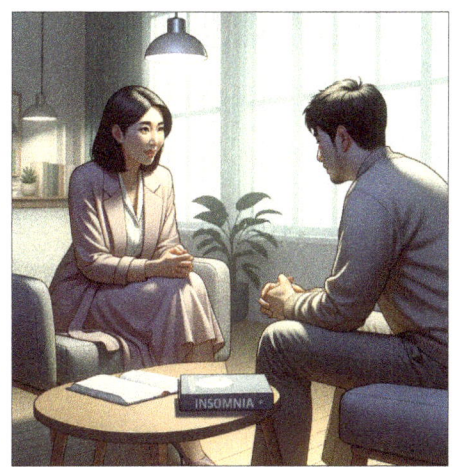

Introduction

This chapter explores the ethical foundations of client education, focusing on the critical role of mutual understanding and compassion in clinical conversations. While the "Theory of Communicative Action" by Jürgen Habermas illuminates the importance of dialogue in social structures, its essence is deeply relevant beyond the academic sphere, particularly in the personalized setting of client education.

Habermas's concept of "lifeworlds" stresses the critical need to appreciate the unique context of a client's life to effectively mitigate personal distress like insomnia. Patient educators can thus calibrate their strategies with precision, ensuring that interventions are intimately attuned to the client's individual experiences and values. This approach safeguards against the intrusion of external pressures, such as societal expectations of healthy sleep and media influence on adopting certain remedies, which can skew the authenticity of the client's lived experience.

This personalized approach will create meaningful insomnia education plans that are aligned specifically to the client's identity and daily life. A commitment to an ethical interaction respects the individual narratives of our clients and seeks to empower them as active participants in their own care.

In the intimacy of the patient educator-client relationship, this approach takes on a therapeutic dimension, offering a unique understanding of each client's condition. It is a testament to the power of empathy in clinical practice, where every conversation is a step towards a more empathic and healthful relationship. Our focus, therefore, is not solely on the scholarly merits of communicative, motivational, and cognitive theories but on their practical application in fostering a compassionate, ethical, and effective client education process.

Clinical Interviewing as the Path to Personalized Plans

The art of clinical interviewing serves as a bridge to deeper understanding. This concept finds resonance in the work of Carl Rogers, the luminary of client-centered therapy. Rogers ardently believed in the power of genuine, empathetic listening, emphasizing the need to set aside personal biases and create an environment of unconditional positive regard. Achieving this internal tranquility is paramount.

By curbing our instinctive rush to advise and filtering out personal predispositions, we pave the way for our clients to narrate their journeys, illuminating their distinctive insomnia challenges. In our program's inaugural session, the clinical interview emerges as a cornerstone. The depth of this engagement dictates the ambiance for subsequent interactions. While active listening may seem unobtrusive, it requires an unwavering commitment and presence.

While there is an innate professional desire to offer immediate solutions, patience is vital. Hastiness can create barriers, preventing clients from opening up. Our goal is insightful companionship, not hasty salvation. This approach ensures we are well-equipped to craft education plans that resonate deeply with each client's narrative.

Maintaining balance is key. While the client's voice remains central, guiding the conversation towards goal-oriented insights is our responsibility.

Deep Listening in Insomnia Assessment

Understanding the Importance of the 'Longform' Approach

- **Drawing parallels to the podcast world:** Just as longform podcasts allow for a thorough exploration of a topic, giving listeners a deep dive into the subject matter, our 'longform' clinical interview approach encourages clients to open up, ensuring nothing is missed.

- *Example: Imagine a podcast episode where the host rushes the guest, cutting off meaningful stories. The audience misses out. Similarly, rushing our clients might mean missing essential insights.*
- **Benefits of a prolonged initial session:** Investing time in the first session provides the depth needed to uncover nuanced insights into a client's insomnia journey, ensuring a solid foundation for subsequent sessions.
  - *Example: Client: "At first, it was just the stress from work. But over time, even on vacations, I found myself restless." Educator: "So, this isn't just about daily stresses; it's evolved over time."*

Preparing for the Interview

- **Crafting the ideal environment:** An inviting, calm space ensures clients feel at ease. A room with comfortable seating, muted colors, and soft lighting can create an atmosphere conducive to open conversation about insomnia.
- **Setting intentions:** It's essential to enter the session with a clear goal. For the educator, it's about understanding; for the client, it's about being understood and finding a solution.
  - *Example: "Today, our primary goal is to understand your sleep journey, Jane. Feel free to share anything you believe is relevant."*

Starting Strong: Initiating the Conversation

- **Opening lines:** These set the tone. Begin with welcoming words that make the client feel valued and understood.
  - *Example: "Welcome, Jane. I appreciate you taking the time today. Let's work together to understand your sleep challenges."*
- **Encouraging client lead:** Give clients the reins initially. This autonomy fosters trust and ensures their most pressing concerns come to the forefront.
  - *Example: Client: "It's been years of restless nights…" Educator: "Tell me more about when it began and what you've experienced."*

The Delicate Art of Note-taking
- **Importance of capturing actual words:** Using the client's own words in notes ensures their feelings and experiences are accurately represented.
- **Introducing note-taking:** By explaining the reason for taking notes and seeking permission, clients feel respected.
  - *Example: "Jane, I'll jot down some notes to ensure I capture everything correctly. Is that alright?"*
- **Tactful note-taking techniques:** The key is being discreet. Avoid long periods of writing, which can disrupt the conversation's flow.

Deep Listening and Reflective Responses
- **Resisting directive questioning:** Let the client's narrative unfold naturally without leading them down a predetermined path.
- **Significance of paraphrasing:** This technique showcases active listening, ensuring the client feels heard.
  - **The Simple Paraphrase:** Rephrase what the client says without altering the message's essence.
    - *Example: Client: "I dread nighttime now." Educator: "Nighttime has become a source of anxiety for you."*
  - **Active Reflection:** This goes a step further, diving into the underlying emotions or thoughts.
    - *Example: Client: "Coffee is my lifeline these days." Educator: "It sounds like you're relying on coffee to cope with the fatigue."*
- **Navigating the complexities of reflective listening:** Sometimes, there might be misinterpretations. It's crucial to adjust and realign based on client feedback.
  - *Example: Educator: "So, work is the primary stressor affecting your sleep?" Client: "Not just work, family issues too." Educator: "Got it, both work and family challenges are impacting your rest."*

Engaging without Intruding
- **Striking the balance:** It's about being a present listener without dominating the conversation or overshadowing the client's voice.
- **Avoiding premature solutions:** Jumping to conclusions can hinder understanding. It's essential to fully grasp the client's experience before suggesting solutions.

Clarifying and Confirming
- **When to seek clarity:** If something is ambiguous, it's better to clarify immediately rather than make assumptions.
  - *Example: Client: "Some nights are just…hard." Educator: "Can you help me understand what 'hard' means for you on those nights?"*
- **Validating feelings and perceptions:** Affirming the client's feelings builds rapport and trust.
- Example: "It sounds incredibly challenging, Jane. Your feelings are valid, and I'm here to help."

Concluding the Interview
- **Summarizing key takeaways:** Briefly recap the primary insights from the session to ensure both parties are on the same page.
- **Setting expectations for session two:** Give a glimpse of the next steps, building anticipation and ensuring the client knows what to expect.
  - *"Today, we've explored your sleep challenges, Jane. In our next session, we'll discuss the insomnia plan I'll craft based on what you've shared with me today."*

Tailored Sample Queries for Insomnia Contexts

In the evolving landscape of patient education, mastering the art of inquiry is both an art and a necessity. Every question we present is important to lay the foundation for their personalized insomnia education plan. The goal isn't just about amassing data; it's about fully understanding and valuing the myriad facets of an individual's life. The subsequent probing questions aim to tap into the various spheres of a client's life, offering educators an enriched perspective. From understanding their emotional triggers to decoding daily routines, these inquiries guide us in crafting tailored strategies for effective insomnia management.

1. **Emotional and Psychological Well-being:**
   - How would you describe your current stress levels, and what are the primary sources of that stress?
   - Are there specific thoughts or worries that frequently occupy your mind, especially before bedtime?
   - Have you ever experienced a traumatic event that you believe might be affecting your sleep?
   - Are there moments from your past that you find yourself thinking about frequently, especially during the night?
   - How would you describe your overall mood and emotional well-being, especially in the evening?
   - Have you noticed any patterns between your emotional state and your sleep quality?

2. **Daily Life and Routine:**
   - Describe a typical day for you, from the moment you wake up to when you go to bed.
   - Can you walk me through your typical evening routine before bed?
   - What are your most cherished daily rituals or habits? Are there any you think might impact your sleep?
   - How do you wind down in the evening before bed?

3. **Relationships and Social Interactions:**
   - How would you describe your relationships with family and friends? Are there any relationships that might be affecting your sleep?

- How do those closest to you describe your sleep habits?
- Do any family members or close friends experience sleep issues? If so, how have they managed or addressed them?
- How often do you engage in social activities? Do you feel these are rejuvenating or draining?
- How does your sleep pattern affect your relationships and daily interactions with others?

4. **Work and Responsibilities:**
   - Tell me about your current job or daily responsibilities. Do you find them fulfilling?
   - How does your daily workload or job responsibilities impact your stress levels and sleep?
   - Have there been significant changes in your work environment or responsibilities lately?

5. **Health and Wellness:**
   - Are there any medical conditions or medications that you believe impact your sleep?
   - Tell me about your diet and exercise routines. Have you noticed any patterns between what you eat or your physical activity and your sleep quality?
   - Do you engage in any recreational substances (like alcohol, nicotine, or caffeine)? How often and in what quantities?

6. **Past Therapies or Treatments:**
   - Have you sought any form of treatment or therapy for your insomnia in the past?
   - What interventions or remedies have you tried in the past for your sleep issues? How did they work for you?
   - Are there any therapies or treatments you're particularly interested in or hesitant about?

7. **Beliefs and Values:**
   - Are there any cultural, spiritual, or personal beliefs that influence your perspective on sleep?
   - How do you define a "good night's sleep"? What does that look like for you?
8. **Change and Adaptability:**
   - Can you recall the last time you made a significant change in your lifestyle or a habit? Who in your life, if anyone, helped you make those changes?
   - How do you generally approach and adapt to changes in your life?

Every individual's story is replete with nuances and layers. Their responses offer more than just answers; they open up gateways into their worlds, highlighting both challenges and strengths. As patient educators, these insights form the bedrock upon which we build their personalized insomnia education plan. The true essence of impactful education interweaves our clinical expertise with the wisdom extracted from these meaningful dialogues. By actively listening and intricately tailoring our interventions to resonate with each client's unique narrative, we not only cultivate trust but also catalyze sustainable improvements in their sleep quality.

CHAPTER 4

Part 2–Building The Data-Informed Client Education Plan

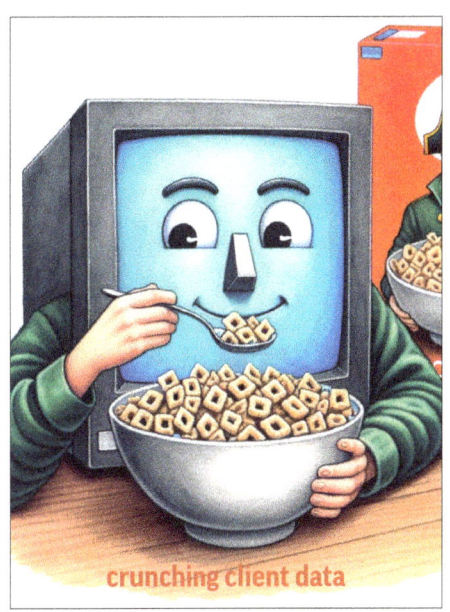

crunching client data

Introduction

As patient educators, we occupy a key role: we listen, analyze, and construct. The essence of our craft is not unlike that of a seasoned computer, where each piece of shared information is a data point feeding into an intricate system of algorithms. In this chapter, we explore the profound responsibility and skill involved in being a confident listener—a mental computer of sorts—capable of crunching numbers, discerning patterns, and building actionable strategies for those grappling with insomnia.

We are the architects of these plans, our neural networks are laden with remedies and insights, aligning each client's unique circumstances with the most suitable interventions. This alignment considers potential resistance areas and cognitive distortions, allowing us to aid our clients in restructuring these thought patterns. Additionally, our understanding of client motivation, quantified by the Insomnia Motivation Inventory (IMI) scores, further refines our computational process, guiding us toward a plan that not only resonates with the client but is also feasible for them to adopt.

Education plans should adapt to client preferences, with options ranging from printed materials for the literary-inclined to interactive digital presentations for dynamic engagement. Employing visual aids and personalized elements, the aim is to deliver a customized, comprehensible, and resonant roadmap to better sleep health.

Data Synthesis: The Mental Computation

In sleep medicine, where sleep's deeply personal nature often makes it a sensitive topic, active listening allows the patient educator to perform a type of mental computation, synthesizing data from the disparate threads of a client's narrative. To aid in this complex task, patient educators should consider utilizing strategic note-taking. This can involve a dual-column method where one side captures direct quotes or key phrases from the client, and the other side notes the educator's observations or interpretations. This allows the educator to remain engaged while ensuring that critical information is recorded. Additionally, employing shorthand symbols or notations can streamline the process, making the review of notes more efficient post-session.

It's also beneficial to periodically summarize the conversation, both to reinforce understanding and to give the client space to correct or expand upon the information shared. The objective is to collect as much data as possible, which may mean creating a visual flowchart of the client's life, sleep patterns, and list of potential contributing factors to their insomnia, which can later be used to generate targeted educational interventions.

How the Insomnia Motivation Inventory (IMI) Affects Which Remedies to Suggest

Behavior change is a multifaceted and dynamic process, often depicted as progressing through stages that include precontemplation, contemplation, preparation, action, maintenance, and relapse. Each stage represents a different level of readiness to commit to change, and our clients' progression through these stages is rarely linear, often moving in a cyclical or spiral manner. This dynamic nature of change underscores the importance of assessing where a client currently stands in their willingness to engage with different insomnia remedies.

The Insomnia Motivation Inventory (IMI) is instrumental in mapping this readiness. By evaluating a client's motivation levels across various domains, we can predict how likely they are to initiate and adhere to a particular intervention. High IMI scores in areas such as Interest/Enjoyment and Perceived Competence suggest that the client may be more inclined to embrace complex remedies that require sustained effort and engagement, such as Clinical and Therapeutic Methods or Traditional Eastern Remedies.

Conversely, lower IMI scores, especially in the Effort or Value/Usefulness subscales, may indicate a preference for or greater success with solutions that demand less initial and ongoing input, like Natural Aids and Supplements or Environmental Adjustments. This understanding allows us to create a hierarchy of interventions, prioritizing them from those requiring high motivation and effort to those that are less demanding.

The IMI scores thus become a lighthouse, guiding the construction of the educational plan. A higher motivation score indicates a readiness to undertake even the most demanding of insomnia remedies, while a lower score suggests a need for interventions that demand less initial effort from the client. Consequently, the educational plan must mirror these scores, starting from the less demanding interventions and progressing towards more intensive ones as motivation increases.

For instance, clients with lower IMI scores may benefit from starting with Environmental Adjustments and Supplementary Aids, which require minimal ongoing effort after initial setup. As their motivation and engagement with the education process grow, they might then be introduced to Lifestyle Hacks and Natural Aids, which necessitate a greater commitment to habit change or product selection. Ultimately, those who express high motivation and readiness for change may find themselves well-suited for Clinical and Therapeutic Methods, as well as engaging in Traditional Eastern Remedies, which call for a significant investment of time and effort in professional guidance and personal practice.

First Look at What's Trending in Insomnia Remedies

In the context of crafting a client's educational plan, the preview of trending insomnia remedies is akin to a curated exhibit where each item is meticulously selected for its relevance and potential impact. This selection must be concise, avoiding an overwhelming array of options, and instead offering a customized collection that harmonizes with the individual's unique profile and motivational readiness as assessed by the Insomnia Motivation Inventory (IMI) scores.

It's crucial to acknowledge that these categories are not absolute—what may require substantial effort for one individual may be less demanding for another, underscoring the importance of personalization. The remedies are presented in a suggested order based on the commitment they typically require, from those necessitating the most effort and motivation to the least. This hierarchy is flexible and adapts to each client's unique situation, ensuring that options are not only effective but also realistically aligned with their current level of engagement and capacity for change. The goal is to ease clients into the client education process, beginning with approaches that match their initial motivation and gradually introducing more demanding strategies as their commitment to improving sleep health strengthens.

Effort-Aligned Insomnia Remedy Rankings

1. **Clinical and Therapeutic Methods**: These methods might include psychotherapy, require a commitment to multiple sessions, sometimes extended over a long period of time, and may involve medical professionals, medications, in-depth analysis, or specialized tools.
2. **Traditional Eastern Remedies**: While some aspects of Eastern practices like acupressure might be self-administered, many, such as acupuncture or certain yoga techniques, require professional guidance and consistent effort to realize benefits.
3. **Mindful Practices**: Establishing a routine or practice around meditation, guided imagery, or progressive muscle relaxation requires dedication, time, and often guidance or training.
4. **Digital Age Solutions**: While some apps may be 'set and forget', many require consistent interaction or data input to be effective. Podcasts for relaxation need active listening, at least initially.
5. **Lifestyle Hacks**: Adjusting exercise routines, managing caffeine, and setting consistent bedtimes involve modifying daily habits which might require consistent effort initially but can become second nature over time.

6. **Natural Aids and Supplements**: These largely involve consumption or application of natural products. While they might require research and trial-and-error to find the right product or dosage, the effort is generally limited to the consumption/application itself.
7. **Environmental Adjustments**: After the initial setup or adjustment (e.g., getting the right mattress, setting up a white noise machine, or adjusting room temperature), these remedies often run in the background and don't require daily effort.
8. **Supplementary Aids**: This category is probably the easiest in terms of effort. Once you've acquired items like weighted blankets, blue light blocking glasses, or earplugs, the effort is just in using them.

Creative Presentation of the Education Plan

Designing the Paper Plan: Aesthetic and Function When constructing the paper plan, it's essential to marry aesthetic appeal with practical functionality. The design should not only be visually pleasing, encouraging clients to engage with the material, but also organized in a manner that facilitates understanding and retention. Utilization of whitespace, clear headings, and bullet points can aid in digesting information. Moreover, the plan should be adapted to individual learning styles, incorporating diagrams or flowcharts for visual learners, and succinct summaries for those who prefer text.

Crafting an Engaging PowerPoint: Tips for Dynamic Interaction An effective PowerPoint presentation for client education transcends static slides and bullet points. To craft a compelling narrative, integrate elements such as relevant storytelling, client-centered scenarios, and interactive questions that invite participation. Slide transitions and animations should be used sparingly to emphasize key points without causing distraction. Furthermore, including short video clips or sound bites can provide a multimodal educational experience, fostering a dynamic learning environment.

Utilizing Visual Aids: Enhancing Plan Comprehension and Engagement Visual aids are instrumental in bridging the gap between complex concepts and client understanding. They can transform abstract ideas into tangible representations, making the education plan more accessible. Charts, models, and infographics can serve as focal points for discussion, sparking curiosity and facilitating deeper understanding. Moreover, visual aids can act as mnemonic devices, assisting clients in recalling important information long after the conversation has ended.

The Use of Color Coding: Organizational and Memory Aids Incorporating color coding within the education plan serves multiple purposes. It provides a visually stimulating experience and operates as an organizational tool, guiding clients through different sections with ease. Each color can represent a distinct theme or concept, thereby aiding in memory retention. For instance, warm colors can denote action items or strategies, while cool colors might highlight background information or relaxation techniques. This method can significantly enhance the learning experience and foster long-term adherence to the education plan.

In an era where digital literacy is ascending, it is crucial to acknowledge that each of these mediums can be adapted for digital consumption. Transitioning from paper to screen, the design principles of the paper plan can be reimagined for digital interfaces, enhancing accessibility and interactivity. Digital documents can be rich with hyperlinks, allowing for an exploratory approach where clients can click through to delve into topics of interest. Similarly, PowerPoint presentations gain a new dimension online; live polls and interactive elements can be embedded, inviting real-time engagement from clients.

Visual aids, too, gain an extended reach in the digital realm. Interactive infographics and clickable charts provide clients with the autonomy to navigate their educational journey at their own pace. Color coding can be adapted for screen use with interactive elements that highlight and expand upon selection, ensuring that the organizational and mnemonic benefits translate seamlessly to the digital environment.

Embracing digital does not merely replicate the paper experience; it enriches it, offering tools for customization and personalization that cater to the unique learning curves of each client. In doing so, the education plan becomes a living document, one that can evolve alongside the client's progress and needs.

CHAPTER 5

Part 3–The Final Clinical Conversation

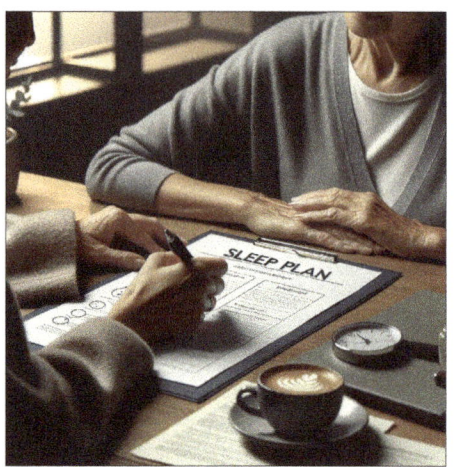

Presenting the Tailored Plan
Instructions to the Patient Educator
- **Ensure both you and the client have a printed copy of the education plan.**
  - Begin the session by handing your client their copy of the education plan. It's important that both of you have a physical copy to refer to during the discussion. This creates a tangible reference point for both parties, allowing for a more focused and meaningful conversation.
  - **Example:** You might start by saying, "Here's your personalized sleep plan. Let's go through this together. Feel free to ask questions or share your thoughts as we move along."
- **Encourage the client to use a pen to mark the plan as you discuss it. This interaction fosters a sense of ownership and makes the plan more personalized.**
  - Urge your client to actively participate in the session by using a pen to highlight or note areas in the plan that stand out to them. This active participation not only helps them to internalize the information but also gives them a sense of control and ownership over their sleep health journey.
  - Example: "Feel free to mark any part of the plan that resonates with you or where you have questions. It's important that this plan feels like it's truly yours. I will mark the same areas so I know what your final plan looks like."
  - Note on presentation medium: Of course, if you are presenting this plan digitally you can edit live as you go. For example if you are sharing your

screen on ZOOM, the edits will be made and the final plan can be resent to your client in real time.

- **Guide the client through each section, allowing them to voice their thoughts and make suggestions. This ensures the plan resonates with their individual needs and preferences.**
  - Take a collaborative approach by inviting your client to express their opinions and suggestions as you walk through each section of the plan. Their input can provide invaluable insights into their personal preferences and lifestyle, allowing for a more effective plan.
  - Example: After explaining a section, ask, "How do you feel about this approach? Are there any adjustments that you think we should make?"
- **Highlight the key elements of the plan, explaining how each part is designed to address specific aspects of their insomnia situation.**
  - Emphasize the critical elements of the plan, detailing how each has been carefully chosen to address particular aspects of the client's insomnia gleaned from the first meeting.
  - Example: "This section here on rearranging your bedroom was designed to help you with the light and noise you told me about in your home around the time you want to get to sleep."
- **Remember, this is likely your final session with the client, so ensure they understand each element of the plan and feel confident in its execution.**
  - Given that this might be the last formal session with the client, it is crucial to ensure they leave feeling confident and well-equipped to implement the plan. Encourage questions and clarify any uncertainties. Reiterate your availability for future support if needed.
  - Example: "I want to make sure you leave today feeling confident about this plan. Please ask any questions you have now. Remember, you can always reach out if something comes up as you start implementing the plan."

Wrapping Up the Session: Empowering the Client for Immediate Implementation

This section aims at concluding the session on a motivational note, equipping the client with practical and immediate steps to begin their journey towards better sleep. It stresses the importance of a positive mindset and the effectiveness of starting with small, manageable changes, setting the stage for immediate action and long-term success.

Instructions to the Patient Educator

- By providing clear, actionable steps that the client can take immediately to start implementing their plan, one of the best gifts you can give to your client is to help them visualize what will happen that very night. Pick one of the easiest recommendations from the plan and tell them how this could easily be implemented in just a few hours, that is, tonight! If one of your recommendations is finding a soothing podcast, they can jump on their phone this evening and find one to try out.
    - Choose a simple, achievable step from their plan that can be initiated right away. This immediate action can build momentum and confidence in their ability to make changes.
    - Example: "Tonight, let's start with something straightforward. How about finding a soothing podcast to listen to as you wind down? It's a small step, but it can make a big difference in setting the tone for your night."
- **Discuss the importance of a positive mindset and how it can significantly impact the effectiveness of the plan.**
    - Emphasize the role of a positive outlook in implementing the plan. Encourage the client to believe in their ability to make changes and improve their sleep health.
    - Example: "A positive mindset is crucial as you start this journey. Believe in the changes you're making and know that each step, no matter how small, is moving you towards better sleep."

- **Encourage the client to start small, focusing on one or two changes to begin with, and gradually incorporate more elements of the plan.**
    - Advise the client to avoid feeling overwhelmed by trying to implement everything at once. Suggest starting with a couple of manageable changes and then gradually adding more.
    - Example: "Let's focus on one or two changes first. Once you feel comfortable with these, we can look at integrating more elements from your plan. This gradual approach can lead to more sustainable changes."

Scheduling Follow-up and Ongoing Support
Instructions to the Patient Educator
- Scheduling Follow-up and Ongoing Support is tricky because in theory this is your last scheduled session with your client, so even though discussing the importance of tweaking the plan as they go is crucial, having the support and feedback of the Patient Educator may or may not be available. This discussion of support will largely depend on the level of motivation and readiness for change the client possesses.
    - It's essential to address the nuances of ongoing support with the client. Explain that while this session might mark the end of scheduled meetings, their journey towards better sleep health is ongoing.
    - Example: "Today might be our last scheduled session, but that doesn't mean your journey ends here. We'll discuss how you can continue to tweak and adapt your sleep plan."
- **Emphasize that check-ins with friends and family are opportunities to solidify their commitment.**
    - Encourage your client to engage their support network. Remind them that sharing their progress and challenges with friends and family can provide additional motivation and accountability.

- Example: "Keeping your loved ones in the loop about your sleep health journey can be incredibly supportive. They can be your cheerleaders and help keep you on track."
- **Clearly outline the support framework available to the client after this conversation. This might include access to online resources, support groups, or periodic check-ins via phone, email, or text.**
    - Provide a list of available resources and explain how each can be beneficial. Emphasize the availability of different forms of support, such as digital resources or community groups.
    - Example: "Apart from our sessions, you have a wealth of resources at your fingertips. Online forums, support groups, and our educational materials can offer additional guidance."
- **Set up a tentative follow-up session, if they desire one, but regardless, reach out via email or text after about a week to see how they are doing, and offer a session if they want one.**
    - Discuss the option of a follow-up session, emphasizing that it's available if needed. Also, commit to reaching out after a week to check on their progress.
    - Example: "Would you like to schedule a follow-up session? Whether or not we do, I'll send a message next week to see how things are going with your new sleep routine."
- **Reinforce the message that the client's journey towards better sleep health is a continuous process and that you are there to support them.**
    - Conclude by reaffirming your commitment to their journey. Make sure they understand that support is ongoing, even if formal sessions are not scheduled.
    - Example: "Remember, improving your sleep is a continuous journey. I'm here to support you, so don't hesitate to reach out if you need guidance or have questions in the future."

This section builds on the importance of ongoing support and provides practical advice for patient educators on facilitating continuous engagement and support for client's post-education plan. It emphasizes the role of external support networks and the availability of various resources while maintaining a focus on the individualized needs of each client.

When Your Client Does Not Want to Say Goodbye
Instructions to the Patient Educator
- Address the possibility of extending sessions, based on the client's needs and progress. In my practice, I will continue to see the client if they so desire. I use a sliding self-pay scale if insurance will not cover the sessions. Many patient educators at medical practices can bill using the ICD code under patient education that works nicely.
    - When a client expresses a desire to continue the sessions, assess their needs and progress to determine if extended sessions would be beneficial. Be prepared to discuss alternative payment options, such as a sliding self-pay scale, especially in cases where insurance may not provide coverage.
    - Example: "If you feel that continuing our sessions would be beneficial, we can certainly explore that option. Let's discuss what that might look like, including how we can manage it financially."
- While it is important to be transparent in discussing your organization's policy regarding extended sessions, follow-up care, and billing, reframe the talk in an empowering way to avoid any perceptions they won't get the support they need from you.
    - It's crucial to communicate your organization's policies clearly but also to reassure the client that their needs and support are your priority. When discussing policies, focus on how these options are designed to empower and support the client's journey.
    - Example: "While we have certain policies for extended sessions and follow-up care, I want you to know that these are in place to ensure you get the

most effective support tailored to your needs. Let's talk about how we can make this work for you."

In this section, the focus is on guiding patient educators on how to handle situations where clients wish to continue their sessions beyond the initially planned duration. It includes practical advice on discussing extended sessions, addressing financial considerations, and framing conversations in an empowering manner to reassure clients about continued support.

"One More Thing Before You Go"– Give Your Clients A Heads Up On Cognitive Distortions

This parting piece of education can make or break the client's progress; it's that powerful. Emphasize to clients that while cognitive distortions and negative self-talk are common, especially at the start of their sleep journey, they can be managed and overcome with practice and the right strategies.

Refer to the comprehensive listing of cognitive distortions and restructuring examples in the following pages by co-occurring disorders, or lifestyle circumstances exacerbating your client's insomnia.

Instructions to the Patient Educator
1. **Educating Clients About Common Cognitive Distortions:**
   - Begin by introducing the concept of 'negative self-talk' or cognitive distortions, focusing on how these irrational thought patterns can negatively impact sleep.
   - Highlight typical distortions such as catastrophic thinking ("If I don't sleep well tonight, I won't be able to function tomorrow") and overgeneralization ("I always sleep poorly, so tonight will be no different").
   - Explain that these thoughts are common, especially in the early stages of implementing a new sleep plan.

2. **Techniques to Recognize and Challenge Distortions:**
   - Teach clients to identify when they are engaging in negative self-talk or distorted thinking.
   - Introduce cognitive restructuring, explaining how to challenge and replace irrational thoughts with more balanced, realistic ones.
   - Encourage clients to question the evidence behind their negative thoughts and consider alternative, more positive perspectives.
3. **Strategies for Combating Negative Self-Talk:**
   - Suggest practical exercises such as thought tracking through journaling, where clients write down their negative thoughts and analyze them for distortions.
   - Offer cognitive restructuring exercises, guiding clients on how to counteract negative thoughts with rational, positive ones.
   - Emphasize the importance of regular practice to develop these skills.
4. **Addressing Common Cognitive Issues Related to Insomnia:**
   - Discuss the link between insomnia and issues like anxiety or maladaptive thinking patterns.
   - Provide strategies to approach these issues, such as mindfulness exercises which can help clients stay present and reduce anxiety.
   - Highlight the normalcy of experiencing mental challenges while adapting to a new sleep routine and the importance of persistence and mental resilience.

Cognitive Distortions in Diverse Insomnia Contexts

Cognitive distortions are ingrained thinking habits that can contribute to emotional distress and reinforce problematic behavior patterns. Combining various sources, including scholarly works and popular self-help literature, here's a comprehensive list of cognitive distortions, simplified for clarity, with explanations and examples. Each distortion is a particular way of viewing the world and oneself, often leading to unnecessary emotional distress or behavioral issues.

- **Insomnia with Shiftwork**
- **Insomnia with PTSD**
- **Insomnia with Anxiety**
- **Insomnia with Depression**
- **Insomnia with Obstructive Sleep Apnea**
- **Insomnia with Bipolarity**
- **Insomnia with Medication-Induced Insomnia**

Insomnia With Shiftwork

This structure helps shift workers recognize and challenge their cognitive distortions, aiding in their adaptation to unusual sleep schedules and improving their overall well-being.

1. Polarized (All-or-Nothing) Thinking
   - Distortion: "If I can't sleep for a full 8 hours, it's as bad as not sleeping at all."
   - Cognitive Restructuring: "Even shorter periods of sleep can be restorative. Quality matters more than strict duration."
2. Jumping to Conclusions

   a. Mind Reading
   - Distortion: "Everyone thinks I'm lazy because I'm tired after a night shift."
   - Cognitive Restructuring: "I can't know what others think. My tiredness is a natural response to shift work, not a reflection of laziness."

   b. Fortune Telling
   - Distortion: "I will never be able to adjust to this shift work."
   - Cognitive Restructuring: "Adjustment takes time. With strategies and patience, I can adapt to this new schedule."
3. Emotional Reasoning
   - Distortion: "I feel so exhausted; it means I'm not cut out for shift work."
   - Cognitive Restructuring: "Feeling exhausted is a normal response to schedule changes. It doesn't mean I can't eventually adapt."

4. Overgeneralization
   - Distortion: "I couldn't sleep well after my last night shift; I'll never be able to adjust to this schedule."
   - Cognitive Restructuring: "One bad night doesn't predict the future. Sleep patterns can improve with time and practice."
5. Labeling and Mislabeling
   - Distortion: "Because I struggle with shift work, I must be weaker than others."
   - Cognitive Restructuring: "Struggling with a challenging schedule is not a reflection of weakness. Everyone has their own adaptation process."
6. Catastrophizing and Minimizing
   - Distortion: "If I don't get a good night's sleep today, my entire week will be ruined."
   - Cognitive Restructuring: "One night's sleep doesn't determine the success of my whole week. I can find ways to cope and recover."
7. Personalization and Blame
   - Distortion: "It's my fault that I'm having trouble adjusting to this shift pattern."
   - Cognitive Restructuring: "Adjusting to shift work is challenging and not solely within my control. Blame is not a constructive response."
8. Should Statements
   - Distortion: "I should be able to sleep anytime if I'm really tired."
   - Cognitive Restructuring: "Sleep is influenced by many factors, not just tiredness. I will find strategies that work for me."
9. Mental Filtering
   - Distortion: "I only remember the bad nights of sleep, not the good ones."
   - Cognitive Restructuring: "Acknowledging both good and bad sleep experiences gives a more balanced view of my situation."

10. Disqualifying the Positive
    - Distortion: "Even when I sleep well, it doesn't matter because I often sleep poorly."
    - Cognitive Restructuring: "Good sleep nights are important and show that positive change is possible."
11. Always Being Right
    - Distortion: "My way of coping with shift work is the only correct one."
    - Cognitive Restructuring: "Being open to different strategies and viewpoints can enhance my ability to cope with shift work."
12. Fallacy of Change
    - Distortion: "My partner or coworkers should adjust their behavior to accommodate my sleep schedule."
    - Cognitive Restructuring: "While support is helpful, expecting others to change for me is not realistic. I can communicate my needs and work on my own coping strategies."
13. Gratitude Traps
    - Distortion: "I shouldn't feel tired or complain because others have it worse."
    - Cognitive Restructuring: "It's okay to acknowledge my own struggles with shift work, even if others have different challenges."

Insomnia with PTSD

Individuals with PTSD often face unique challenges in achieving restful sleep, primarily due to the lingering psychological impacts of their trauma. This section explores common cognitive distortions in those suffering from PTSD-related insomnia, alongside strategies for cognitive restructuring. By understanding and addressing these specific thought patterns, clients can learn to manage their sleep difficulties more effectively, fostering a healthier sleep environment and a more positive mindset.

1. **Catastrophizing**: Imagining the worst-case scenarios related to an event or situation.
   - *Distortion*: "If I have a nightmare tonight, it means I'm regressing in my healing."
   - *Cognitive Restructuring*: "One nightmare does not define my overall progress. Healing is a journey with ups and downs."
2. **Hyper-Vigilance to Threat**: Always being on the lookout for danger, even in safe environments.
   - *Distortion*: "If I go to sleep, something bad might happen."
   - *Cognitive Restructuring*: "I am in a safe environment now. Sleep is a natural and necessary process, and it's okay to let my guard down."
3. **Overgeneralization**: Believing that because they experienced trauma once, they're doomed to experience it again.
   - *Distortion*: "Every noise at night is a threat."
   - *Cognitive Restructuring*: "Not every noise is a sign of danger. Some sounds are just a normal part of the environment."
4. **Emotional Reasoning**: Allowing emotions to drive interpretation of reality.
   - *Distortion*: "I feel terrified right now; it means I'm in danger."
   - *Cognitive Restructuring*: "Feelings are not always facts. Just because I feel scared doesn't mean there's an immediate threat."
5. **Personalization**: Feeling personally responsible for the traumatic event or its aftermath.
   - *Distortion*: "It's my fault I can't sleep; I should be over this by now."
   - *Cognitive Restructuring*: "Healing is a unique process for everyone. My struggles with sleep are a reaction to trauma, not a personal failure."
6. **Selective Abstraction**: Focusing on a single negative detail and ignoring the positives or the bigger picture.
   - *Distortion*: "I woke up once last night; my therapy isn't working."

- *Cognitive Restructuring*: "Progress in therapy isn't linear. One restless night doesn't negate the other nights of improvement."
7. **Mental Filtering**: Focusing excessively on negative events and discounting positive ones.
    - *Distortion*: "I had a good week of sleep, but last night was bad, so things are getting worse again."
    - *Cognitive Restructuring*: "One bad night doesn't erase the progress I've made. It's okay to have setbacks; they don't define my entire journey."

Insomnia with Anxiety

People diagnosed with anxiety often have specific cognitive distortions that impact their sleep patterns. Here's a structured breakdown:

1. **Catastrophizing**: Imagining and fearing the worst possible outcome, especially about future events.
    - *Distortion*: "If I don't sleep well tonight, I'll mess up everything tomorrow and people will judge me."
    - *Cognitive Restructuring*: "One restless night doesn't determine my entire day. Even if tomorrow is challenging, I have faced challenges before and persevered."
2. **Overgeneralization**: Drawing a broad conclusion from a single or few events.
    - *Distortion*: "I always struggle to sleep before big days. I'll never overcome this."
    - *Cognitive Restructuring*: "While I've had challenges, there have been times I've slept better than expected. Each night is a new opportunity."
3. **Fortune Telling**: Predicting events will turn out badly without evidence.
    - *Distortion*: "I just know I won't be able to fall asleep tonight because I'm feeling anxious."
    - *Cognitive Restructuring*: "I can't predict the future. While I'm feeling anxious now, it's possible for me to relax and have a restful night."

4. **Labeling**: Assigning labels to oneself based on perceived shortcomings.
   - *Distortion*: "I'm such a failure because I can't manage a basic thing like sleep."
   - *Cognitive Restructuring*: "Everyone has challenges. Struggling with sleep doesn't define my worth or capabilities."
5. **Magnification and Minimization**: Exaggerating negatives and understating positives.
   - *Distortion*: "I woke up multiple times last night, so my entire sleep was worthless."
   - *Cognitive Restructuring*: "While I did wake up, there were also periods I slept soundly. Some rest is better than none."
6. **Personalization**: Believing that one is the cause of external events.
   - *Distortion*: "My partner seems tired; it's my fault because I kept tossing and turning."
   - *Cognitive Restructuring*: "There are many reasons someone could be tired. I shouldn't automatically assume responsibility for others' feelings."
7. **What If Questions**: Continually asking "what if" about future negative events, leading to more anxiety.
   - *Distortion*: "What if I can't fall asleep tonight? What if that leads to health problems?"
   - *Cognitive Restructuring*: "Engaging in 'what ifs' only increases my anxiety. I will focus on the present and the steps I can take now for better sleep."

Insomnia with Depression

Depression can introduce its own set of cognitive distortions which can further complicate sleep challenges. Understanding these cognitive distortions is essential when working with insomnia sufferers with depression. Addressing and challenging these distortions using cbt-i and behavioral therapy approaches can have a meaningful impact on their sleep and overall mental health.

Here's the structured breakdown for insomnia sufferers with a depression diagnosis:

1. **Catastrophizing**: Viewing or presenting a situation as considerably worse than it actually is.
   - *Distortion*: "This one bad night of sleep is proof that my life is spiraling out of control."
   - *Cognitive Restructuring*: "Everyone has off nights. One bad sleep doesn't mean everything is falling apart."
2. **Overgeneralization**: Making a broad conclusion based on a single event.
   - *Distortion*: "I had trouble sleeping last night; I'll never have a good night's sleep again."
   - *Cognitive Restructuring*: "Sleep patterns can vary. One restless night doesn't predict every future night."
3. **Filtering (Selective Abstraction)**: Focusing entirely on negative elements of a situation and filtering out positive ones.
   - *Distortion*: "I woke up a few times during the night, so it was a terrible sleep."
   - *Cognitive Restructuring*: "While I did wake up, there were stretches when I slept deeply. I should acknowledge the whole picture."
4. **All-or-Nothing Thinking (Polarized Thinking)**: Viewing situations in black-and-white, with no middle ground.
   - *Distortion*: "I didn't get a full 8 hours; my sleep was a complete waste."
   - *Cognitive Restructuring*: "Quality matters more than exact quantity. Some solid rest is still beneficial."
5. **Personalization**: Taking personal responsibility for things that are outside of one's control.
   - *Distortion*: "It rained and I had a bad sleep; it's my fault for not having a better environment."
   - *Cognitive Restructuring*: "There are factors, like the weather, that are beyond my control. I did the best I could with what I had."

6. **Helplessness**: Believing that one has no control over situations in their life.
   - *Distortion*: "There's no point in trying sleep aids or techniques; nothing will help."
   - *Cognitive Restructuring*: "There are many strategies and aids I haven't tried. It's worth exploring options to improve my sleep."
7. **Emotional Reasoning**: Believing that the way one feels reflects reality.
   - *Distortion*: "I feel hopeless about my sleep situation, so it must be hopeless."
   - *Cognitive Restructuring*: "My feelings are valid, but they don't always paint the full picture. There are paths to better sleep that I can pursue."

Insomnia with Obstructive Sleep Apnea

Obstructive Sleep Apnea (OSA) can have significant effects on an individual's sleep quality and lead to specific cognitive distortions due to the nature of the condition. Here's the structured breakdown for insomnia sufferers with OSA:

1. **Catastrophizing**: Magnifying the negative implications of their sleep disorder.
   - *Distortion*: "Because I have OSA, I'll never experience a good night's sleep again."
   - *Cognitive Restructuring*: "With the right treatment and adjustments, I can manage my OSA and improve my sleep quality."
   - *Distortion*: "If my CPAP machine makes a noise tonight, I'll never get any sleep."
   - *Cognitive Restructuring*: "Adjustments can be made, and one noisy night doesn't mean every night will be disrupted."
2. **Overgeneralization**: Drawing broad conclusions from a single incident or symptom.
   - *Distortion*: "I felt tired today, so my CPAP therapy must not be working at all."
   - *Cognitive Restructuring*: "There can be various reasons for feeling tired. I shouldn't rush to conclusions based on one day."

- *Distortion*: "I felt claustrophobic with the mask once; I'll never be able to tolerate it."
- *Cognitive Restructuring*: "Comfort with the mask can vary. I might feel differently with adjustments or over time."

3. **All-or-Nothing Thinking (Polarized Thinking)**: Believing that if sleep isn't perfect, then it's a complete failure.
   - *Distortion*: "If I can't use my CPAP every single night, there's no point in having it."
   - *Cognitive Restructuring*: "Consistent use is important, but missing one night doesn't negate its overall benefits."
4. **Labeling**: Assigning negative labels to oneself based on their medical condition.
   - *Distortion*: "I have OSA; I'm a broken sleeper."
   - *Cognitive Restructuring*: "Having OSA is a medical condition, not a reflection of my worth or identity. It's something I'm managing."
5. **Personalization**: Blaming oneself for the development of OSA or related challenges.
   - *Distortion*: "It's my fault I developed OSA."
   - *Cognitive Restructuring*: "There are many factors, including genetics and physical structure, that contribute to OSA. It's not a matter of personal fault."
6. **Helplessness**: Believing there's no hope for improvement or change.
   - *Distortion*: "No matter what treatment I try, my OSA won't get better."
   - *Cognitive Restructuring*: "There are various treatments and interventions available. With the right guidance and persistence, I can find what works best for me."
7. **Filtering (Selective Abstraction)**: Focusing solely on the negative aspects of OSA and ignoring any positive progress.
   - *Distortion*: "Even with the CPAP machine, I had a brief awakening last night. The treatment is useless."

- *Cognitive Restructuring*: "While I might still have occasional awakenings, the CPAP has reduced many of the severe symptoms of OSA."
8. **Minimization**: Underplaying the significance or effectiveness of positive events or strategies.
    - *Distortion*: "Sure, the CPAP helps a bit, but it's not making a big difference."
    - *Cognitive Restructuring*: "Every bit of improved sleep quality counts. Recognizing the benefits can motivate consistent use."

Insomnia with Bipolarity

It's paramount for insomnia sufferers with bipolar disorder to recognize these cognitive distortions. With the ebbs and flows of mood in bipolar disorder, consistent sleep is a pillar of stability. Properly addressing these distortions in therapy can aid in achieving better sleep and mood management.

1. **Catastrophizing**: Magnifying the negative implications of a situation.
    - *Distortion*: "If I can't sleep tonight, it might trigger a manic episode and everything will fall apart."
    - *Cognitive Restructuring*: "While sleep is important for managing my mood, one restless night doesn't determine my entire mood trajectory. I have strategies to cope."
2. **Overgeneralization**: Extending one instance to predict a consistent pattern.
    - *Distortion*: "I've had insomnia during my last manic phase; I'll always struggle with sleep during such phases."
    - *Cognitive Restructuring*: "Each episode and its symptoms can vary. I can learn and apply strategies to improve my sleep."
3. **Personalization**: Believing events or reactions of others are a direct response to one's actions or characteristics.
    - *Distortion*: "My partner looks tired; it's because I kept them up with my insomnia."

- *Cognitive Restructuring*: "Everyone can have off days. I shouldn't assume it's always connected to me or my sleep patterns."

4. **All-or-Nothing Thinking (Polarized Thinking)**: Viewing situations only in black and white.
   - *Distortion*: "If I don't get a full night's sleep, it's completely worthless."
   - *Cognitive Restructuring*: "Some rest is better than none. Even brief periods of sleep can be rejuvenating."

5. **Emotional Reasoning**: Believing feelings are a direct reflection of reality.
   - *Distortion*: "I feel like I won't sleep tonight, so it's bound to happen."
   - *Cognitive Restructuring*: "My feelings are a response to many factors, and while they're valid, they don't predict the future. I can take steps to relax."

6. **Magnification of Positives (during manic/hypomanic episodes)**: Overestimating the positives of not sleeping.
   - *Distortion*: "Not sleeping gives me more time to be productive and creative!"
   - *Cognitive Restructuring*: "While I might feel a surge of energy, consistent sleep is crucial for my well-being and mental stability."

7. **Mind Reading**: Assuming to know what others think without concrete evidence.
   - *Distortion*: "Everyone can tell I didn't sleep well and they think less of me for it."
   - *Cognitive Restructuring*: "I can't know for sure what others are thinking. Everyone has off days and most are focused on their own experiences."

Insomnia with Medication-Induced Insomnia

Many medications can have side effects that lead to insomnia. Patients who are aware of these side effects might develop cognitive distortions related to their medication and its impact on their sleep. Here's the structured breakdown:

1. **Catastrophizing**: Overestimating the negative impact of a situation.
   - *Distortion*: "If this medication disrupts my sleep, it's going to ruin my health and life."
   - *Cognitive Restructuring*: "While the medication might affect my sleep, there are strategies I can employ to manage and mitigate its effects."
2. **Overgeneralization**: Assuming that a single event's outcome will always be the same in future occurrences.
   - *Distortion*: "I couldn't sleep well the first night of taking the medication; it will always affect me this way."
   - *Cognitive Restructuring*: "The body often adjusts to new medications over time. One restless night doesn't predict every future night."
3. **Personalization**: Feeling that the insomnia is a personal failing rather than a side effect.
   - *Distortion*: "Other people can handle this medication without problems; there must be something wrong with me."
   - *Cognitive Restructuring*: "Everyone's body reacts differently to medications. It's not a reflection of my worth or strength."
4. **All-or-Nothing Thinking (Polarized Thinking)**: Viewing situations only in black and white.
   - *Distortion*: "If the medication causes insomnia, I have to stop taking it entirely."
   - *Cognitive Restructuring*: "There might be ways to manage the side effect or adjust the dosage. I should consult with my doctor before making decisions."
5. **Emotional Reasoning**: Taking feelings as a direct reflection of reality.
   - *Distortion*: "I feel like this medication will cause me to never sleep well again."
   - *Cognitive Restructuring*: "Feelings aren't always facts. While I'm concerned, it's essential to see how the medication affects me over time."

6. **Filtering (Selective Abstraction)**: Focusing only on the negative aspects and ignoring the positive.
   - *Distortion*: "This medication helps my condition, but the sleeplessness is all I can think about."
   - *Cognitive Restructuring*: "While managing the side effect is important, I should also acknowledge the benefits the medication brings."
7. **Jumping to Conclusions**: Making a prediction based on little to no evidence.
   - *Distortion*: "I read online that someone couldn't sleep because of this medication, so I'm sure it will happen to me."
   - *Cognitive Restructuring*: "Everyone's experience with a medication is unique. I should monitor my own reactions and consult with my healthcare provider."

CHAPTER 6

The Spectrum of Modern Insomnia Remedies

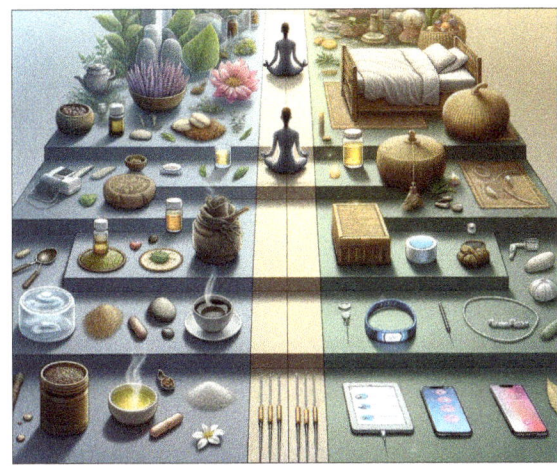

In your role as a patient educator, the clinical conversations provide the necessary context to identify the most suitable remedy for each client, acknowledging their unique experiences and needs. This spectrum of remedies ranges from traditional practices like acupuncture to contemporary solutions such as digital sleep-tracking apps. Consider this chapter as an essential part of your toolkit, bridging the gap between the rich insights gained from clinical interviews and actionable, effective solutions.

As you navigate through this extensive list, remember not to be overwhelmed by the variety of options. Instead, refer back to your notes from clinical conversations and trust your intuition to guide you. The journey to achieving restful sleep is often complex and non-linear, resisting any standardized fix. It demands a thoughtful combination of various approaches. Utilize this comprehensive list, presented in alphabetical order in the following pages, as a foundation to inform and enhance your collaborative journey with clients towards achieving restorative sleep. Your discernment and intuition are key in selecting the right combination of remedies for each individual client.

Insomnia Remedies Alphabetized

1. **4-7-8 Breathing**: A controlled breathing technique that may mitigate stress when mindfulness meditation does not suffice. It involves a rhythmic pattern of inhaling for four seconds, holding the breath for seven seconds, and exhaling for eight seconds, potentially enhancing relaxation.

2. **Acupressure**: A non-invasive intervention derived from Traditional Chinese Medicine, employing manual pressure to specific meridian points to alleviate insomnia symptoms by restoring energy balance.
3. **Acupuncture**: This ancient Chinese medicinal practice inserts fine needles into the skin at strategic points, potentially modulating neuroendocrine activity and fostering a state of relaxation that can alleviate insomnia.

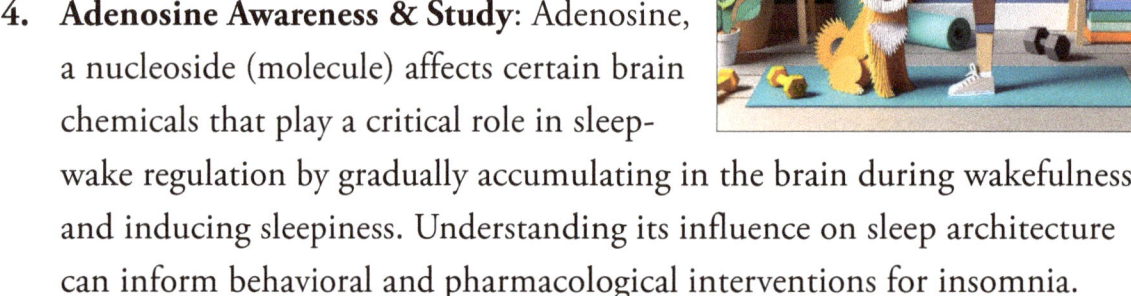

4. **Adenosine Awareness & Study**: Adenosine, a nucleoside (molecule) affects certain brain chemicals that play a critical role in sleep-wake regulation by gradually accumulating in the brain during wakefulness and inducing sleepiness. Understanding its influence on sleep architecture can inform behavioral and pharmacological interventions for insomnia.
5. **Aerobic Exercise Timing**: Engaging in aerobic exercise can elevate body temperature and stimulate the hypothalamic-pituitary-adrenal axis, leading to increased alertness. Timing exercise in the late afternoon allows for the subsequent reduction in core body temperature and cortisol levels, which may facilitate sleep onset.

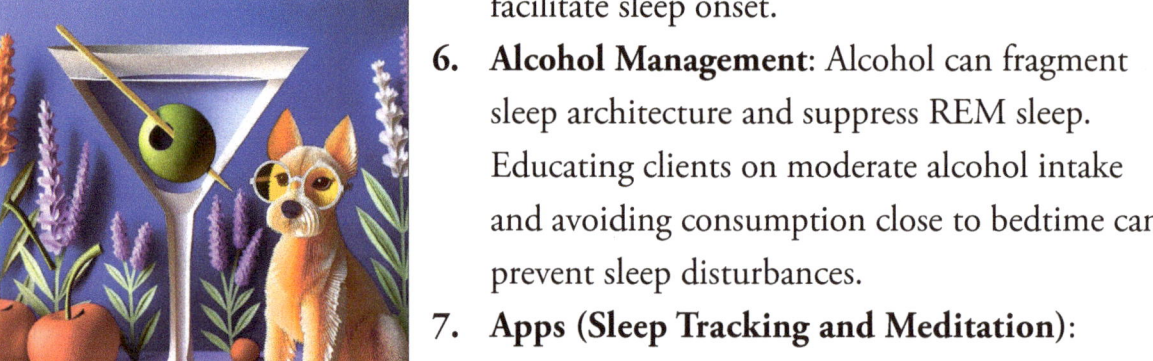

6. **Alcohol Management**: Alcohol can fragment sleep architecture and suppress REM sleep. Educating clients on moderate alcohol intake and avoiding consumption close to bedtime can prevent sleep disturbances.
7. **Apps (Sleep Tracking and Meditation)**: These digital applications can provide valuable feedback on sleep patterns or facilitate pre-sleep

relaxation through guided meditation, potentially improving sleep hygiene and onset latency.

8. **Aromatherapy**: The inhalation of essential oils, such as lavender or chamomile, may exert anxiolytic and sedative effects, possibly through the modulation of GABAergic neurotransmission, which can be conducive to sleep.
9. **Bedtime Consistency**: Maintaining a consistent sleep schedule can synchronize the circadian rhythm with the external environment, optimizing the timing of melatonin secretion and enhancing sleep quality.
10. **Blue Light Blocking Glasses**: These glasses can attenuate blue light exposure from electronic devices, which may otherwise suppress nocturnal melatonin production and delay sleep onset.
11. **CBD Oil or Edibles**: Cannabidiol has been hypothesized to exert anxiolytic effects through its action on the endocannabinoid system, potentially reducing sleep latency and nocturnal awakenings.
12. **Cherry Juice (Tart Cherry)**: Contains natural melatonin and anthocyanins, which may have sleep-enhancing properties by improving the availability of tryptophan and modulating inflammation.
13. **Chinese Dietary Practices**: Traditional Chinese dietary principles focus on the balance of "qi" and blood, with certain foods believed to have properties that can promote sleep by nourishing the heart and calming the mind.
14. **Clock Watching**: Obsessive time-checking can increase stress and perpetuate a cycle of sleep anxiety. Advising clients to turn clocks away can help reduce preoccupation with sleep duration.
15. **Cognitive Behavioral Therapy (CBT) for Insomnia**: A structured program that addresses cognitive and behavioral factors contributing to insomnia, with evidence supporting its efficacy in improving sleep parameters.

16. **Consistent Room Temperature**: The thermal environment can influence sleep quality. A slightly cool room temperature aligns with the body's nocturnal temperature dip and can facilitate the onset of sleep.
17. **Deep Breathing**: Slow, diaphragmatic breathing may activate the parasympathetic nervous system, reducing sympathetic arousal and promoting relaxation conducive to sleep.
18. **Dietary Caffeine Management**: Caffeine is a well-known stimulant that can prolong sleep latency and impair sleep quality. Advising clients on limiting caffeine intake, particularly in the hours before bedtime, can be beneficial.

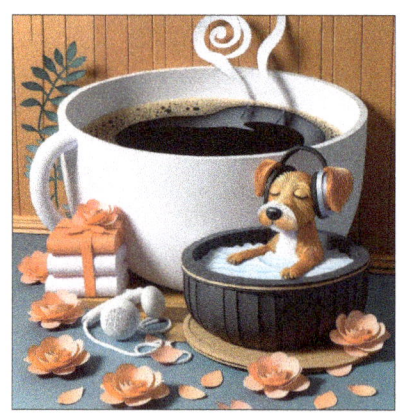

19. **Earplugs**: Use of earplugs can attenuate environmental noise, which is especially beneficial for individuals with heightened auditory arousal during sleep.
20. **Essential Oils (like Lavender)**: Certain essential oils are posited to have sedative properties that may facilitate relaxation and improve sleep quality through olfactory stimulation.
21. **Exercise**: Regular physical activity has been associated with deeper sleep stages and improved sleep continuity, although the timing of exercise relative to bedtime is crucial to avoid counterproductive arousal.
22. **Foot Soak and Reflexology**: The practice of soaking feet in warm water and applying reflexology may induce relaxation through warm temperature and tactile stimulation, potentially easing the transition to sleep.
23. **Guided Imagery**: This relaxation technique involves the mental visualization of calming images or scenarios, which may reduce cognitive arousal and facilitate sleep onset.
24. **Herbal Supplements (e.g., Valerian Root, Melatonin)**: These supplements contain compounds that may influence sleep through various biological

pathways, although their efficacy and mechanism of action can vary among individuals.

25. **Hot Baths or Showers**: The post-bath drop in body temperature can mimic the natural decline in core temperature that occurs during sleep onset, potentially signaling the body that it is time to sleep.
26. **Hot Yoga**: The combination of yoga poses with a heated environment can enhance relaxation and reduce stress, potentially improving sleep quality.
27. **Hypnosis**: Hypnotherapy may facilitate sleep by inducing a state of deep relaxation and altering sleep-related cognitions.
28. **Journaling**: The act of writing down thoughts and concerns before bedtime can help in the cognitive processing of daytime stressors, potentially reducing rumination and facilitating sleep.
29. **Light Therapy**: Exposure to bright light at specific times can shift the phase of the circadian rhythm, beneficial for individuals with circadian rhythm sleep-wake disorders.
30. **Machines (White Noise, Sound Machines)**: These devices can create a consistent auditory backdrop that may mask disruptive environmental sounds, promoting uninterrupted sleep.
31. **Massage Therapy**: Massage can reduce physical tension and promote relaxation through the manipulation of soft tissues, which may have beneficial effects on sleep quality.
32. **Mattresses**: An ergonomically designed mattress can provide appropriate support for the body, which is essential for maintaining comfort and spinal alignment during sleep, potentially reducing awakenings and improving sleep quality.
33. **Meditation**: Mindfulness meditation can decrease cognitive and physiological arousal, which may be beneficial for individuals with insomnia.
34. **Medication*** (Prescription and Over-the-Counter Sleep Aids): Pharmacological agents can be used to induce or maintain sleep, although they may have side effects and risks of dependence.

35. **Mouth Tape**: Taping the mouth shut to encourage nasal breathing can improve sleep quality and reduce snoring by optimizing airflow during sleep.
36. **Music Therapy**: Listening to calming music can lower stress and anxiety levels, which may be conducive to sleep induction.

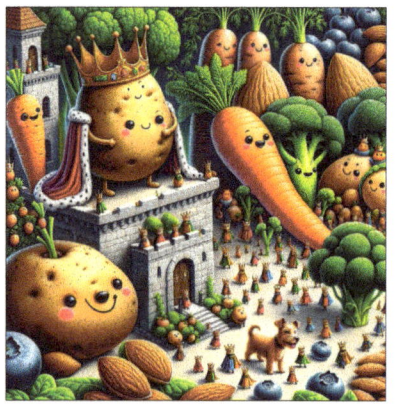

37. **Nap Management**: Strategic napping can be beneficial for individuals with sleep onset difficulties, provided that naps are short and not too close to bedtime.
38. **Nose Tape**: Similar to mouth tape, nose tape can improve nasal airflow, which may be beneficial for sleep, particularly in individuals with certain respiratory conditions.
39. **Nutrition**: A balanced diet that avoids large meals, caffeine, and alcohol before bedtime can positively influence sleep quality.
40. **Podcasts**: Listening to relaxation-focused podcasts can provide a narrative distraction that may facilitate the transition to sleep.
41. **Progressive Muscle Relaxation**: This technique involves sequentially tensing and relaxing muscle groups, which may reduce somatic tension and promote a state conducive to sleep.
42. **Psychoanalysis**: This therapeutic approach explores underlying psychological conflicts, which may contribute to insomnia, particularly when psychodynamic factors are at play.
43. **Reading**: Engaging with a physical book before bedtime can be a relaxing activity that distracts from daily stressors and prepares the mind for sleep.
44. **Relaxation Techniques (like Visualization)**: These techniques can reduce anxiety and tension, potentially improving sleep quality by promoting a state of mental and physical calm.
45. **Sex**: Sexual activity can have a sedative effect, possibly due to the release of endorphins and oxytocin, which may promote relaxation and sleepiness.

46. **Sleep Clinics**: Specialized centers that provide diagnostic evaluation and treatment for sleep disorders, offering a range of therapeutic interventions.
47. **Sleep Diaries**: The systematic recording of sleep-related information can help identify patterns and behaviors that may contribute to insomnia.
48. **Sleep Scheduling**: Establishing a regular sleep-wake schedule can reinforce the circadian rhythm and improve sleep efficiency.
49. **Sleep Restriction**: This behavioral technique limits the amount of time spent in bed to the actual sleep time, which can consolidate sleep and increase sleep drive.
50. **Sleep Retreats**: These programs offer a combination of sleep-promoting activities and therapies in a tranquil environment, which may be beneficial for individuals with insomnia.
51. **Tea (Herbal, like Chamomile)**: Certain herbal teas contain compounds with potential sedative effects that may calm the nervous system and promote sleep.
52. **Temperature Control**: Regulating the bedroom temperature to maintain a cool environment can facilitate the body's natural thermoregulatory processes during sleep.
53. **Tryptophan-rich Snacks**: Consuming foods high in tryptophan before bedtime can increase the availability of this amino acid for serotonin and melatonin synthesis, which may promote sleepiness.
54. **Weighted Blankets**: These blankets apply gentle, even pressure across the body, which may reduce anxiety and create a sense of security, potentially improving sleep quality.
55. **Worry Time and Journaling**: This strategy involves setting aside a specific period earlier in the evening for clients to engage in 'worry journaling'—the process of writing down concerns and anxieties. By transferring thoughts from mind to paper, clients can contain their worries within this designated

timeframe, which can prevent rumination at bedtime. This practice not only helps in organizing thoughts and identifying patterns but also provides a psychological buffer to separate the day's stressors from the sleep period, potentially improving sleep onset and quality.

56. **Yoga**: The practice of yoga combines physical postures, breathing exercises, and meditation, which may reduce stress and promote relaxation conducive to sleep.

57. **Yoga Nidra**: Also known as "yogic sleep," this guided meditation technique induces a state of deep relaxation while maintaining consciousness, which may be beneficial for individuals with insomnia.

*Regarding prescription medications: While the direct management of pharmacological treatments is outside the scope of a patient educator's role, providing support and education about potential side effects and the importance of adherence to prescribed regimens is crucial. This support is part of the collaborative effort to ensure comprehensive care for clients with insomnia.

CHAPTER 7

Insomnia: Five Case Studies

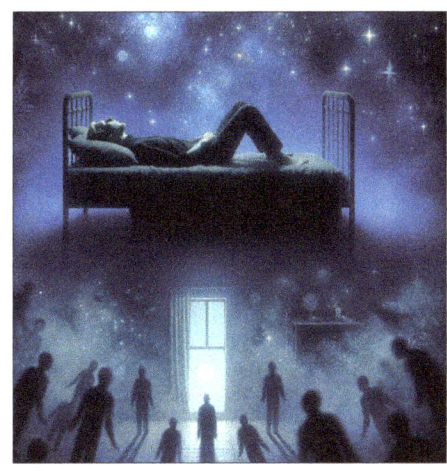

In the U.S., chronic insomnia affects about 10–30% of adults, with higher rates among women and older adults over 60, linked to hormonal changes and age-related health shifts. Notably, young people increasingly experience insomnia due to a unique blend of stress, including academic and social pressures, future employment concerns, and the impact of constant digital connectivity.

There is a significant association between insomnia and mental health disorders. Conditions such as anxiety and depression are commonly found in individuals with insomnia, with evidence suggesting a bidirectional relationship where each condition can exacerbate the other. Additionally, chronic illnesses, including chronic pain, diabetes, heart disease, and respiratory disorders, are correlated with higher rates of insomnia. Socioeconomic factors significantly influence insomnia prevalence, with individuals under economic and social stress, especially those with lower incomes or employment-related stress, more prone to developing insomnia.

As we navigate the broad spectrum of insomnia's impact, it becomes clear that behind each statistic lies a personal story, a unique struggle with sleep. This chapter unfolds the narratives of five distinct individuals, each exemplifying a unique aspect of insomnia and its diverse impact on people from all walks of life. Our journey begins with Janice, a seasoned teacher whose nocturnal worries about work, family, and her own sense of self-worth have ensnared her in a relentless cycle of sleeplessness. We then meet Anthony, a night-shift security guard whose irregular schedule and personal stressors have culminated in a disrupted circadian rhythm. Ria, a young art student, grapples with her gender identity, cultural pressures, and anxiety, all of which weave into her intricate tapestry of insomnia.

In addition to Janice, Anthony, and Ria, we explore the stories of Hannah and Joe, each bringing unique perspectives to the complex world of insomnia. Hannah, a 66-year-old retiree in Nashville, confronts the dual challenge of chronic back pain and lingering insomnia following opioid misuse. Her journey reveals the intricacies of managing sleep disorders in the golden years, accentuating the influence of physical health and environment on sleep quality.

Joe's story takes us to San Antonio, where as an Iraq War veteran, he faces a nightly battle with PTSD-triggered insomnia. His struggle highlights the profound impact of past traumas on sleep and the complex interplay between mental health and lifestyle choices.

The aim of presenting these case studies is twofold. Firstly, it is to illuminate the diverse ways insomnia manifests in individuals' lives, influenced by factors such as age, lifestyle, past experiences, and mental health. Secondly, it is to showcase how patient education, shaped by the unique complexities of each case, can pave the path to better sleep and, consequently, an improved quality of life.

Disclaimer

The case studies presented in this chapter are hypothetical scenarios, carefully crafted for educational purposes. They are not derived from any specific individual client encounters but instead are composites, amalgamating a range of symptoms, situations, and experiences that have been observed in clinical practice over many years.

Furthermore, the therapeutic approaches, interventions, and recommendations discussed in relation to these case studies are based on a combination of clinical expertise, current research, and established best practices within the field of sleep medicine. However, they should not be viewed as prescriptive solutions for real-life cases. Each individual experiencing sleep disorders or insomnia has unique needs and should seek personalized advice and treatment from qualified healthcare professionals.

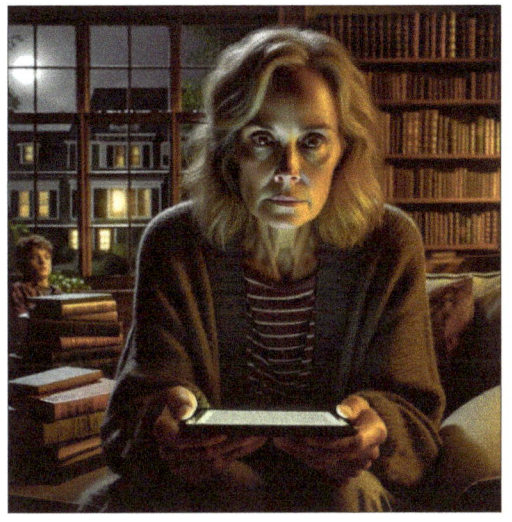

The Tired Teacher

In the quiet town of Lakeview, Wisconsin, Janice, a seasoned high school English teacher, finds herself wrestling with insomnia's cruel grip. At night, her mind becomes a theatre of sorts, replaying scenes from her life—each more vivid than the last. She contemplates her students' futures, wondering if they truly grasp the life lessons embedded in "To Kill a Mockingbird." She worries about her daughter Samantha's adjustment to college life and whether her son Ben is making good choices while out with friends.

Adding complexity to her thoughts is her newfound love for e-books, which she often reads on her tablet late into the night. Despite having a cherished library of first editions just off her living room—a testament to her lifelong love of literature—the allure of instantly accessible digital reads has added another layer to her bedtime routine.

These thoughts spiral into deeper concerns. She begins to question her own teaching methods, asking herself if she's becoming outdated in her pedagogy. Her mind then drifts to her husband Mark, the ever-supportive librarian who curates reading lists for her book club. "Is he happy? Are we growing apart as the kids leave the nest?" she wonders. These racing thoughts, fueled by her vivid imagination and her educator's instinct for constant reflection, leave her lying awake for hours.

Janice's ordeal doesn't end when she finally manages to sleep; she finds herself waking up multiple times. The quality of her sleep is poor, and she wakes up feeling as if she's been in a battle rather than in bed. Her days are tinged with a foggy haze, making her daytime hours as draining as her nights. This cycle has become a self-reinforcing loop; her insomnia feeds her daytime worries, and her daytime worries feed her insomnia.

Last year, Janice was prescribed Zoloft to address a depressive episode. While it helped her mood, it didn't provide the restorative sleep she so desperately craves. Now, her primary focus is breaking free from insomnia's relentless cycle.

Having the Clinical Conversation with Janice

Setting: *A comfortable, softly-lit office with soft chairs and calming artwork on the walls. A small table between the chairs holds a pitcher of water and two glasses. Janice sits across from the patient educator, looking hopeful but a bit apprehensive. The patient educator begins with a warm, encouraging smile.*

Find depth and nuance in Janice's life. Questions that follow serve as a cornerstone for the patient educator to engage in a substantive dialogue with her. These queries aim to explore the multifaceted aspects of Janice's life that might be contributing to her insomnia. It's crucial to bear in mind that the more Janice is willing to share, the more personalized and subsequently effective her education plan will be.

Important Note: While these questions provide a guide for patient educators, it's important to remember that asking all of them in a 2–3 hour session may be too time-consuming. Select questions that naturally fit the conversation's flow for a comprehensive yet focused dialogue.

1. "Janice, can you share more about your evening reading habits? How has the transition from physical books to e-books impacted your bedtime routine?"
2. "It sounds like your children growing up and becoming more independent has had a significant impact on you. Can you describe how the house feels to you now, especially during the evening?"
3. "I noticed you've taken a liking to herbal teas, especially chamomile. How did you come to include this in your evening routine? Have you noticed any changes in your sleep since then?"
4. "Janice, you spend a lot of time pondering over your teaching methods and your students' futures. How does this mental engagement impact your ability to wind down at night?"
5. "Your bond with Mark seems deep. How has he been supporting you through this period? Are there specific instances or conversations that stand out?"

6. "You mentioned feeling like you're in a fog during the day. How does this daytime haze feed back into your insomnia? Are there specific triggers you've identified?"
7. "You have a tendency to reflect deeply, questioning even your own teaching methods. Could you talk about how this constant state of reflection influences your ability to fall asleep?"
8. "You seem very focused on breaking free from this self-reinforcing loop of insomnia and daytime worries. Have you tried any strategies that showed even a glimmer of improvement?"

Building Janice's Education Plan

Upon an in-depth review of the clinical conversation with Janice, it becomes evident that her insomnia is a complex interplay of emotional, environmental, and lifestyle factors. Janice's emotional landscape is particularly compelling, influenced by her children's burgeoning independence and her professional self-doubt. These internal dialogues are further complicated by her transition to e-books, which could be interfering with her circadian rhythm. Given her high IMI scores, we recognize Janice's strong motivation to improve her sleep, which opens the door for a nuanced plan addressing her unique emotional and environmental variables.

Possible Recommendations for Janice's Insomnia Education Plan
Mindful Practices:
Journaling:
- **Recommendation:** Empowering Janice to put her thoughts on paper could serve as a cathartic exercise, helping her disengage from the emotional whirlwind before bedtime.
- **Teaching Method:** A guided journaling session could be the start, where Janice is provided with specific prompts that focus on her concerns. For example, "List three thoughts that frequently keep you awake, and beside each, write an alternative, more positive perspective."

Guided Imagery:
- **Recommendation:** Given Janice's rich literary background, constructing an imagined, peaceful environment drawn from her favorite novels could facilitate a smoother transition to sleep.
- **Teaching Method:** Use an audio guide or a script that incorporates elements from her cherished literary works. Imagine walking through the gardens of Pemberley while narrating the guide in a tone similar to Jane Austen's.

Environmental Adjustments:

Light Therapy:
- **Recommendation:** Light therapy could serve as a strategic intervention to recalibrate her circadian rhythm. This approach holds particular promise during the seasonally darker months.
- **Teaching Method:** A hands-on demo session using a light therapy box, explaining its optimal usage and timing, could be invaluable. You might also discuss how light therapy can align with her teaching schedule.

Natural Aids and Supplements:

Herbal Teas:
- **Recommendation:** Introducing a curated selection of sleep-inducing teas such as valerian root or lavender could serve as a calming ritual before bed.
- **Teaching Method:** A tea-tasting session during which various herbal blends are sampled can make this a fun and educational experience. Discuss the potential sleep benefits of each blend and how she can incorporate them into her evening routine.

Lifestyle Hacks:

Regular Bedtimes:
- **Recommendation:** Implementing a consistent bedtime routine could offer Janice a framework of stability.

- **Teaching Method:** Create a visual bedtime schedule that she can put up in her bedroom. Include time slots for her new rituals like herbal tea and journaling.

Mindful Practices:
- **Journaling**: Empowering Janice to put her thoughts on paper could serve as a cathartic exercise, helping her disengage from the emotional whirlwind before bedtime.
- **Guided Imagery**: Given Janice's rich literary background, constructing an imagined, peaceful environment drawn from her favorite novels could facilitate a smoother transition to sleep.

Natural Aids and Supplements:

Herbal Teas
- **Recommendation:** Introducing a curated selection of sleep-inducing teas such as valerian root or lavender could serve as a calming ritual before bed.
- **Teaching Method:** Provide Janice with a "Tea Menu" handout that lists various herbal teas, their sleep benefits, and optimal brewing instructions. You could also include a small sample pack of teas for her to try at home. During the session, engage her in a conversation about her taste preferences and how she could integrate this ritual into her existing evening routine.

Once the data has been crunched and recommendations are drafted, patient educators have the freedom to get creative in how they present this plan to Janice. Considering that our client is an English teacher with a love for literature, the presentation could employ various forms of media that resonate with her:
- **Paper Plan**: A beautifully printed plan, possibly designed like a book or a thematic brochure that ties into her love for literature.
- **PowerPoint Presentation**: For a more interactive experience, consider building a succinct yet visually engaging PowerPoint that can be walked through together during the session.

- **Visual Aids**: Given Janice's fondness for imagery, consider incorporating illustrations or even quotes from her favorite novels to make the plan more relatable and engaging.
- **Color Coding**: Use colors to highlight different aspects of the plan—Mindful Practices in one hue, Environmental Adjustments in another, etc., making it easier for Janice to digest and refer back to.

Whichever medium you choose, the key is to make the plan as accessible and appealing to Janice as possible. This ensures not just understanding but also emotional engagement, which can be a significant motivator for sticking with the recommendations.

The mode of presentation could, in itself, be a part of the therapeutic alliance you're building with Janice. Your creativity here is not just a formality; it's an extension of the patient education process, further personalizing her experience and potentially enhancing her adherence to the plan.

The Second Conversation with Janice

Setting: *A well-lit room that signifies a fresh start, the atmosphere has been subtly updated since their last meeting. A marker board stands near the plush chairs, ready to visualize key points of the conversation. The patient educator greets her with a familiar affirming smile, signaling they are ready to advance in the next chapter of her sleep education journey.*

Patient Educator: Janice, it's good to see you again. I've spent some time reviewing our notes from our previous session, and I believe I've come up a plan that aligns with your lifestyle and preferences. Would you like to hear what I've come up with?

Janice: Absolutely. I've been looking forward to this.

Patient Educator: Wonderful. First, let's delve into **Mindful Practices**. Given your love for literature, I think you'll benefit from **Guided Imagery**. It's a technique that allows you to visualize calming scenarios, which can help relax the mind and prepare it for sleep. Think of it as reading a story with your mind's eye.

Janice: That sounds intriguing. Like visualizing a scene from a Jane Austen novel?

Patient Educator: Exactly! You have the idea. Next, I'd like you to try **Journaling**. It'll be a space for you to process your feelings, whether about your children's growing independence or past events that have resurfaced.

Janice: I used to keep a journal in college. I think this will be a good way for me to connect with myself again.

Patient Educator: I'm glad to hear that. Now, in terms of **Environmental Adjustments**, I think you'd benefit from **Light Therapy**. Using a light box in the morning can help reset your internal clock. This is especially useful during winter months.

Janice: I've heard of those. Do you think it would help with my late-night reading habit?

Patient Educator: It should. And speaking of reading, I recommend transitioning back to physical books before bedtime. The blue light from electronic devices can interfere with the sleep-wake cycle.

Janice: That's a lot of changes, but they all make sense. And honestly, I miss the feel of physical books.

Patient Educator: Take it one step at a time, and see what resonates with you. I've also noted you've developed a liking for chamomile tea. There are other **Herbal Teas**, like valerian root, known to aid in sleep.

Janice: I'm open to trying. Especially if it means a good night's sleep.

Patient Educator: Lastly, let's talk about **Lifestyle Hacks**. Consistency is key. Establishing **Regular Bedtimes** will help your body recognize when it's time to wind down.

Janice: That's a comprehensive plan. It feels made just for me. I'm ready to give this a shot.

Patient Educator: I'm glad to hear that. Remember, this is a collaborative effort. Work with the plan for two weeks, then we'll meet again to discuss how it's going and make any necessary adjustments. You're not on this journey alone, Janice.
Janice: Thank you. I feel more hopeful than I have in a long time.

Helping Janice with Cognitive Distortions

Navigating the labyrinth of insomnia isn't solely about physical adjustments or environmental tweaks; it's equally about confronting and restructuring the cognitive distortions that exacerbate the sleep issues. For Janice, these distortions are multifaceted—spanning her professional life, personal relationships, and self-perception. By identifying these thought patterns and offering cognitive restructuring techniques, we can empower Janice to challenge her automatic negative thoughts. This is a crucial step in breaking the vicious cycle of daytime worries feeding her insomnia and vice versa. Below, we explore specific distortions Janice is grappling with and provide cognitive restructuring strategies tailored to her context.

1. **Mind Reading in the Classroom:**
    - **Distortion:** "My students probably think I'm a bad teacher because I probably look so tired all the time."
    - **Cognitive Restructuring:** "Students appreciate effort and understanding, not how awake I look. I bring much more to the classroom than just | my appearance."

2. **Catastrophizing Academic Outcomes:**
   - **Distortion:** "Because I couldn't sleep well last night, I'll probably mess up my lesson today, and it'll affect the entire semester."
   - **Cognitive Restructuring:** "One off day doesn't define the entire teaching experience. I have many opportunities to make positive impacts."

3. **Overgeneralization of Feedback:**
   - **Distortion:** "One parent gave me negative feedback about online lessons; this means all parents probably feel I'm not doing enough."
   - **Cognitive Restructuring:** "Different parents have different perspectives. One feedback doesn't encompass the views of all."

4. **Filtering (Selective Abstraction) in Self-Assessment:**
   - **Distortion:** "I struggled with last week's lesson because of my insomnia, so I'm not cut out for this profession."
   - **Cognitive Restructuring:** "I've had countless successful lessons and moments of connection with students. It's essential to consider the broader picture and not just focus on isolated events."

5. **Catastrophizing the gravity of a situation:**
   - **Distortion**: "The silence in this house means I'm alone and will always feel this loneliness."
   - **Cognitive Restructuring**: "The house is quieter, but it also means Samantha and Ben are growing up and finding their paths. They are always a part of my life, even if they're not always present."

6. **Mind Reading by believing to know the thoughts of others without evidence:**
   - **Distortion**: "Mark must be regretting marrying someone like me. I've become such a burden."

- **Cognitive Restructuring**: "Mark has been supportive throughout. I shouldn't assume his feelings based on my insecurities."

7. **Personalization by Taking Personal Responsibility for Someone Else's Behavior:**
   - Distortion: "Samantha hasn't called in days; I must've done something to upset her. Just like I must've instigated the conflict with my colleague."
   - Cognitive Restructuring: "Samantha is in college and might be busy; her silence isn't necessarily a reflection of something I've done wrong. Similarly, the disagreement with my colleague was a two-way interaction that escalated, and it's not solely my responsibility."

Janice's Progress, Setbacks & Recovery

Janice plunged enthusiastically into the patient education process, embracing the array of strategies crafted to her unique needs. Mindful practices like journaling and guided imagery became her outlets for introspection, helping her navigate the emotional complexities tied to her family's dynamics and her own self-doubt in her teaching career.

Within the first month, Janice started to see the benefits of environmental adjustments. Light therapy, particularly useful during the darker winter months, aided in resetting her internal clock. Transitioning back to physical books before bedtime also made a noticeable difference, reducing her exposure to sleep-disrupting blue light. She felt more rested in the classroom, more energetic, and subsequently more confident in her teaching.

However, the path wasn't entirely smooth. Around two months in, Janice encountered a stressful period at school. Increased work responsibilities coincided with a disagreement with a fellow teacher over a shared project. The tension escalated, and Janice lost her temper. This emotional unrest led to a lapse in her newfound habits, notably a return to late-night e-book reading.

Acknowledging this hiccup, Janice scheduled another session with her patient educator. They revisited her progress and pinpointed the triggers leading to this momentary step back. Leaning on her intellect, she modified her journaling to 'worry journaling,' where she would list people and things that weighed heavily on her mind, and by closing the journal would symbolically put them aside and temporarily out of her mind, helping her settle to prepare for sleep.

During the recovery phase, adjustments were made to Janice's plan. Her daytime sleepiness was addressed with a more structured approach to naps, particularly useful after exhausting days at school.

Self-compassion became a focal point in Janice's recovery. The educator reminded her that extending kindness to oneself is vital during setbacks, reinforcing her spiritual beliefs and adding another layer to her emotional resilience.

The subsequent months of Janice's journey narrated a story of transformation. Despite periods of struggle, the overarching theme was one of growth and reconnection with her own needs and potentials. Janice not only managed to navigate the complexities of insomnia but also found a renewed sense of self in the process.

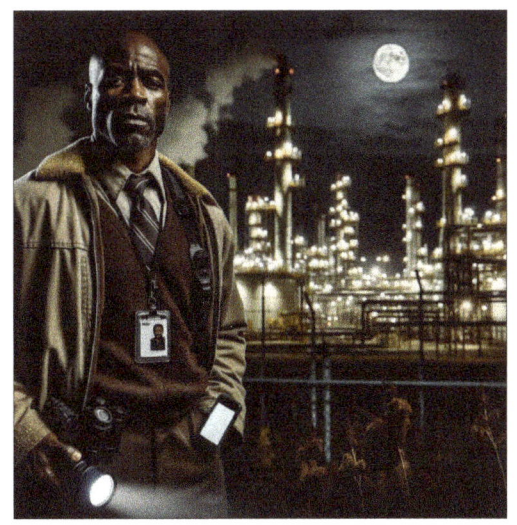

Night Owl Anthony

Anthony, a 35-year-old security guard, has been patrolling a sprawling petrochemical facility from dusk till dawn for the last 10 years. He lives in a small apartment in a Chicago suburb, not too far from the facility. The isolation of his night shifts provides him a sense of peace, but it's also made him a reluctant insomniac. His biological clock seems to be stuck perpetually in "night mode," making the quest for restorative sleep a continual challenge.

Father to two middle school twin boys active in football and baseball, Anthony cherishes the weekends when they visit. However, their youthful energy and late-night escapades further scramble his already erratic sleep pattern. Compounding this is his contentious relationship with his ex-wife, Patricia, who works as a bartender. Their regular spats over money, particularly the soaring costs of the boys' sports activities, serve as a nightly mental preoccupation that keeps him awake.

Anthony is a self-proclaimed "creature of the night," a title he proudly wears as a fan of all genres of movies and television shows, especially space-alien creature films like "War of the Worlds." Sometimes at work he sneaks in a movie on his smartphone while he drinks coffee to stay awake.

A few months back, Anthony had a literal wake-up call. He dozed off during his shift, and a minor system malfunction set off a high-decibel alarm. The moment was heart-stopping. The malfunction could have caused a toxic gas leak, posing a severe risk to the facility and surrounding areas. That jarring moment served as a reality-check about the very real dangers tied to his insomnia, prompting him to finally consult a sleep physician.

Anthony's Intrinsic Motivation Inventory (IMI) scores are low. He's baffled by the idea that achieving quality sleep could require effort. "Why should sleep be work? It's not like hitting the gym," he muses. Coincidentally, the gym has recently become his new playground, as he wants back into the dating scene and wants to 'look good for the ladies'. He's also active on MATCH.com, often excitedly scrolling through potential matches just before trying to sleep, adding yet another hurdle to his already complex journey toward restorative sleep.

Having the Clinical Conversation with Athony

Setting: A well-appointed meeting room within a primary care physician's group office. The room features ergonomic chairs surrounding a round table, with medical literature neatly stacked in one corner. Educational posters about sleep health adorn the walls, and a small potted plant adds a touch of life to the room. Anthony sits across from the patient educator, visibly interested but showing signs of fatigue. The patient educator begins with a warm, encouraging smile.

1. "Anthony, you've been working night shifts for quite some time. How do you generally feel during those hours?"

2. "You mentioned the weekends you spend with your sons. How do you feel those weekends influence your sleep schedule?"
3. "I understand there are financial concerns, especially with your sons' sports activities. Do these concerns ever come to mind as you're trying to get some rest?"
4. "You seem to enjoy movies and TV shows, especially ones with a sci-fi twist. When do you usually find time to indulge in this interest?"
5. "Could you tell me about the incident at work where the alarm went off? How did that experience affect your perspective on your insomnia?"
6. "You scored low on the Intrinsic Motivation Inventory. How do you feel about putting in effort to improve your sleep?"
7. "You've recently taken up going to the gym. How does that fit into your daily routine?"
8. "You mentioned you're active on MATCH.com. How does this activity fit into your evening routine?"

Building Anthony's Education Plan

Anthony's insomnia appears to be a byproduct of a disrupted circadian rhythm, a complex emotional landscape, and lifestyle habits that are counterproductive to restorative sleep. His low IMI scores indicate that any recommendations must be simple to implement and require minimal effort on his part. The plan should address his unique work schedule, his responsibilities as a father, and his interests in movies and physical fitness.

Possible Recommendations for Anthony's Insomnia Education Plan
Lifestyle Hacks:

Caffeine Reduction:
- **Recommendation**: Anthony's coffee consumption is a concern, but let's make it easy. Aim to reduce the amount by just one-third, and shift the last cup an hour earlier than usual.

- **Teaching Method**: Provide Anthony with a simple tracking sheet to log his daily caffeine intake. Point out that this is a moderate adjustment, not an extreme change like halving his coffee intake or quitting cold turkey.

Screen Time:
- **Recommendation**: Instead of action-packed alien movies, Anthony could switch to slower dramas or informative but non-stimulating documentaries. For MATCH.com, recommend scaling down the time spent browsing profiles before bed—starting with 15 minutes, then 10, and finally 5, eventually shifting this activity to his waking hours or work breaks.
- **Teaching Method**: Discuss the idea of stimulus control, focusing on how certain activities can rev up the brain when it's time to wind down.

Environmental Adjustments:

Noise and Light Management:
- **Recommendation**: Given his need for daytime sleep, white noise could help mask daytime noises, and blackout curtains can make his room dark enough for better sleep.
- **Teaching Method**: Share a list of white noise apps or inexpensive white noise machines. If possible, play a few samples during the session. Discuss the benefits of a dark sleep environment, especially during the day, and show him options for blackout curtains.

Financial Worries:
- **Recommendation**: Since financial concerns, particularly regarding his sons' sports, weigh on his mind, a simple financial tracking app might offer some peace.
- **Teaching Method**: Introduce Anthony to a user-friendly budgeting app where he can log expenses. The act of tracking might offer a sense of control, thereby reducing bedtime anxiety over finances.

Given that Anthony is a night shift security guard with a penchant for movies and a low motivation score, the plan presentation should be straightforward and engaging, requiring minimal effort on his part to understand and implement. Here are some tailored presentation ideas:

- Digital Plan: Since Anthony enjoys movies and technology, consider sending him a concise digital plan that he can easily access on his smartphone during breaks.
- Visual Clips: Incorporate short video clips or animations that explain each recommendation. Given his love for visual media, this could be a great way to catch his attention.
- Interactive App: Consider using an interactive mobile app that tracks his sleep habits and caffeine consumption. The app could send timely reminders, making it easier for him to follow the plan.
- Laminated Card: Given his work environment, a small, laminated, pocket-sized card outlining the key recommendations could be practical. He can keep this in his uniform pocket for easy reference.
- Real-life Examples: Use relatable scenarios or anecdotes that tie into his life and responsibilities, such as the importance of sleep for work performance and family life.

Whichever medium is chosen, the goal is to make the plan as accessible and relatable to Anthony as possible. The presentation style is not merely a formality but an essential part of the patient education process. It's about creating a plan that Anthony will not only understand but also feel motivated to follow, despite his initially low motivation levels.

The Second Clinical Conversation with Anthony

Setting: *A professional office space within a medical building. This time, the atmosphere has been subtly changed from their last encounter. A large screen is ready for a PowerPoint presentation, signaling a more formal yet interactive session. The patient educator greets him with an affirming nod, indicating they're ready to move forward in his sleep education journey.*

Patient Educator: Anthony, it's good to see you again. I've been reviewing the information we gathered during our last conversation, and I've tailored a plan that I believe fits your lifestyle and addresses your specific challenges. Would you like to dive in?

Anthony: Sure, let's see what you got.

Patient Educator: Excellent. Let's start with Lifestyle Hacks. I know you consume a lot of coffee during your shifts. I'm not going to ask you to quit cold turkey, but how about we aim to reduce that by one-third?

Anthony: Hmm, that doesn't sound too bad. What's the catch?

Patient Educator: No catch. Just a simple tracking sheet to log your daily caffeine intake and perhaps moving your last cup an hour earlier than usual. Easy, right?

Anthony: Alright, I can try that.

Patient Educator: Great. Next, Screen Time. I know you love your movies, especially the action-packed ones, and you spend time on MATCH.com. Instead of limiting your screen time, how about switching from action-packed films to slower dramas or documentaries closer to bedtime? And maybe limit your MATCH.com scrolling to 15 minutes, then after a week maybe down to 5 minutes on the app. Eventually, I'd like to see you on MATCH after you wake, not just before sleep.

Anthony: That seems doable. But why the change in movie genre?

Patient Educator: Different types of content have different effects on our arousal levels. Slower dramas or documentaries might be less stimulating, helping you wind down. Also, we suggest enabling "night mode" on your devices to reduce blue light exposure.

Anthony: Got it, less stimulation before sleep.

Patient Educator: Exactly. Finally, let's talk about your Environment. Considering you sleep during the day, how about using white noise to drown out daytime noises and installing blackout curtains to mimic nighttime? These blackout curtains on Amazon are both affordable and effective (Patient Educator hands Anthony a printout of the curtains to get him intrigued with the idea).

Anthony: That could work. My apartment does get pretty loud during the day.

Patient Educator: Perfect. So, this is your starting point. Work with the plan for a couple of weeks, and then we'll reconvene to see how things are going. Remember, you're not in this alone, Anthony.

Anthony: Alright, let's do this. But just so you know, I'm doing it for my boys and for the new dates I'll get from MATCH.com.

Patient Educator: Whatever your motivation, it's a step in the right direction. See you in two weeks, Anthony.

Helping Anthony with Cognitive Distortions

Addressing insomnia for Anthony isn't just about cutting back on coffee or screen time; it's also about dealing with cognitive distortions that worsen his sleep issues. Anthony grapples with specific distortions related to his financial worries, work stress, and his role as a parent. Below, we explore these distortions and offer cognitive restructuring strategies.

1. **Financial Catastrophizing:**
   - **Distortion:** "If I can't sleep, I'll perform poorly at work and eventually lose my job. Then, how will I pay for my sons' activities?"

- **Cognitive Restructuring:** "A bad night's sleep is not a predictor of job loss. I have skills and experience that make me valuable at my job."
2. **Overgeneralizing Work Incidents:**
    - **Distortion:** "The alarm incident at work is a sign that I'm not cut out for this job."
    - **Cognitive Restructuring:** "One incident doesn't define my entire career. I've successfully managed many night shifts before."
3. **Parental Guilt:**
    - **Distortion:** "Because I'm tired all the time, I'm probably not being a good dad."
    - **Cognitive Restructuring:** "My worth as a father isn't determined by how many hours of sleep I get. I support my sons in many ways."

Progress, Setbacks & Recovery

Anthony initially approached the patient education process with skepticism but was willing to try for the sake of his sons and potential relationships. While he wasn't enthusiastic about the number of changes he had to make, he was pleased they were relatively easy to implement.

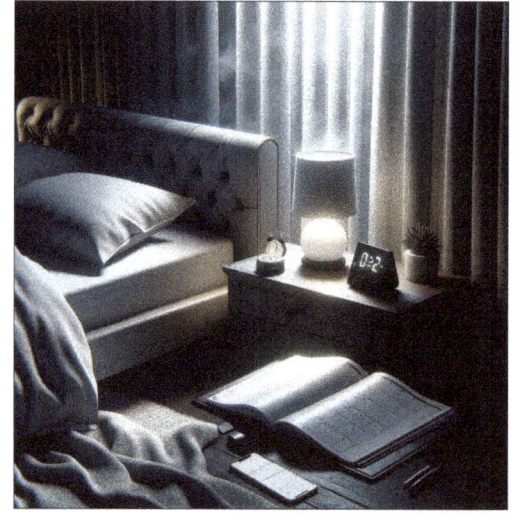

Within the first few weeks, Anthony noticed that he felt less jittery due to the reduction in coffee and that he was falling asleep quicker thanks to changing his viewing habits before bed. Even his day sleep improved with the addition of white noise and blackout curtains, despite the daytime commotion.

However, setbacks were inevitable. A particularly tough week of night shifts and increased responsibilities with his sons led to a relapse in his old habits. Instead of seeing this as a failure, Anthony scheduled another session with his patient educator to recalibrate his plan.

It became clear that Anthony's concerns about money were a recurring issue, so this was incorporated into his cognitive restructuring techniques. The concept of "Progress, Not Perfection" was introduced to him as a way to understand that setbacks are a part of the journey, not an end.

In the following weeks, Anthony made fewer but more impactful changes. His focus shifted to manageable modifications that would still have a significant positive impact on his sleep and overall well-being.

While his journey was not without its bumps, the prevailing theme became one of gradual improvement and increased self-awareness. Anthony realized that the key to better sleep and a better life wasn't just about following a set of rules but about understanding himself more fully and making changes accordingly.

The Nocturnal Art Student

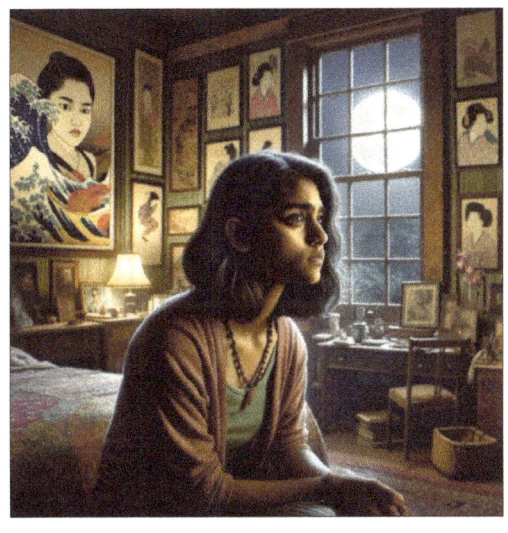

In the picturesque town of Willow Creek, Iowa, Ria finds her nights just as colorful as her days but for all the wrong reasons. This small community, known for its annual arts festival and scenic bike trails, provides a stark contrast to her internal chaos. By day, she's a dedicated barista and a part-time art student, passionate about traditional Japanese art. Her bedroom is a visual treat, adorned with intricate tapestries, and ukiyo-e prints, making it a serene yet vibrant space that reflects her love for art.

She lives in a spacious home with a pool, a place where family gatherings are a common affair. Her father, a cardiologist, and her mother, a homemaker, are originally from Mumbai and have strong traditional beliefs. Recently, they've been in talks with a family from a neighboring town for a possible match for Ria, a prospect that adds another layer of emotional turmoil to her life. While her parents remain blissfully unaware of her gender identity struggles, Ria senses that her siblings are picking up on her emotional disarray, making her family home feel more like a pressure cooker.

Four years ago, Ria was diagnosed with generalized anxiety disorder. She started talk therapy but felt compelled to stop, not because of money but due to the lack of LGBTQ-specific mental health support in her therapy sessions. She even tried anti-anxiety medication briefly but stopped because it made her feel emotionally flat, robbing her of the emotions she channels into her art.

Ria's insomnia is an echo chamber for her complex internal conflicts. She's torn between societal expectations and her own journey of self-discovery concerning her gender identity. Her love for art, while a source of joy, also fuels doubts about her future in an already competitive field. The matchmaking efforts by her traditional family add another layer to her stress, alongside the ever-present specter of generalized anxiety.

During the sleepless nights, her mind becomes an endless loop of these thoughts, each amplifying the other. Despite the ornate beauty of her room and the tranquility it's meant to offer, her nights feel like a never-ending series of anxious thoughts, rather than the restorative sleep she desperately needs.

Ria's Intrinsic Motivation Inventory (IMI) scores are not that high, indicating her hesitation to tackle her sleep issues head-on. She's cautious when it comes to receiving help, wary of any standardized fix that doesn't consider her unique challenges. This leads her to consult a sleep specialist, opening her up to specialized insomnia education that is tailor-made for her complex emotional and mental landscape.

Having the Clinical Conversation with Ria

Setting: *A modern, well-lit consultation room within a primary care physician's group that specializes in sleep disorders. The room features both medical literature and some artwork reflecting diverse cultures, perhaps making Ria feel more at home. Ria sits across from the insomnia educator, her posture a bit closed off but her eyes curious.*

1. **"Ria, you're navigating some complex emotions and thoughts, especially during the night. How is that affecting your daily activities and focus on your art?"**
    a. **Reasoning:** This question invites her to open up about the interaction between her emotional landscape and her insomnia, without directly prying into sensitive issues.
2. **"You stopped talk therapy because it wasn't addressing your specific LGBTQ needs. What are you hoping to gain from this specialized insomnia education?"**
    a. **Reasoning:** This question addresses her past experiences with healthcare, gauging what her expectations and apprehensions might be this time around.
2. **"Your Intrinsic Motivation Inventory scores aren't that high, which tells me you're cautious. What would help you feel more comfortable engaging in this process?"**
    a. **Reasoning:** Given her low IMI scores, this motivational interviewing question seeks to understand her reservations, opening the door to address them directly.
2. **"Ria, tell me about your art practice. How does it fit into your daily life?"**
    a. **Reasoning:** This connects her passion to her sleep patterns, which might reveal if her art-related activities are potential triggers or relievers for her insomnia.
2. **"You've expressed concern about 'standardized fixes.' Could you share what kind of approach you feel would be most beneficial for you?"**
    a. **Reasoning:** This directly addresses her skepticism and provides an opportunity to align the patient education process with her unique needs and expectations.
2. **"What are you looking for in a sleep solution?"**
    a. **Reasoning:** This open-ended question gives Ria the floor to define her own needs and preferences, highly relevant for someone cautious of a standardized fix.

Building Ria's Education Plan

With Ria's low levels of intrinsic motivation and her complex emotional and mental landscape, the educator faces a challenge: to build trust and rapport while also making her feel seen and heard. The aim is to navigate her unique situation without resorting to a standardized fix, all while slowly kindling her motivation to engage more openly in the patient education process.

Ria's insomnia is a multi-faceted issue with a complex interplay of emotional, psychological, and social factors. These range from generalized anxiety disorder to ongoing gender identity struggles and emotional turmoil stemming from traditional family expectations. Her low Intrinsic Motivation Inventory (IMI) scores reveal a sense of caution and reluctance to engage in the patient education process, which is crucial information for an insomnia educator.

Traditional Eastern Remedies:

Yoga & Yoga Nidra:
- **Recommendation:** These could be helpful given their alignment with her interest in Eastern practices.
- **Teaching Method:** Have on hand literature about these practices to alleviate stress and anxiety.

Supplementary Aids:

Weighted Blanket:
- **Recommendation:** Given Ria's love for room decor and her need for emotional comfort, a weighted blanket could offer a sense of security and improve sleep quality.
- **Teaching Method:** Introduce her to the benefits of using a weighted blanket, explaining how the evenly distributed weight can create a feeling of being held, which may help in reducing anxiety and promoting restful sleep.

Natural Aids and Supplements:

CBD Oil:
- **Recommendation:** Given her previous experience with anti-anxiety medications, she might be open to natural alternatives.
- **Teaching Method:** Provide literature on the efficacy of CBD oil for sleep and relaxation.

Environmental Adjustments:

Temperature Control:
- **Recommendation:** Considering her room already offers visual comfort, focusing on optimal temperature might enhance sleep quality.
- **Teaching Method:** Discuss how room temperature can significantly affect sleep quality and suggest ways to achieve the ideal sleep environment.

Mindful Practices:

Color Journaling with Colored Pens:
- **Recommendation:** Since Ria is passionate about art, encourage her to use color journaling as a way to visually represent and process her complex emotions. This creative outlet could be a therapeutic way to offload worries before bedtime, potentially improving her sleep quality.
- **Teaching Method:** Provide her with a blank journal and a set of colored pens. Guide her through the concept of color journaling, where each color could represent a different emotion or worry. The idea is to draw or jot down her worries in a colorful way and then symbolically leave them behind by closing the journal before sleep.

With Ria's low levels of intrinsic motivation and complex emotional terrain, the challenge here is twofold: to foster a sense of trust and to provide education that is as unique as her life experience. The aim is to gently nudge her toward engagement while respecting her individual needs

The Second Conversation with Ria

Setting: *A cozy, art-inspired room within a specialized sleep clinic. The room is decorated with diverse pieces of art making Ria feel more welcomed. Ria walks in, her posture slightly more open than before but still tinged with caution. She sits across from the insomnia educator, who greets her with a warm smile.*

Insomnia Educator: Ria, it's good to see you again. How have you been feeling since our last conversation?

Ria: It's been a mix, but I've been looking forward to seeing what you've come up with for me.

Insomnia Educator: That's what I like to hear! Let's start with Traditional Eastern Remedies. How do you feel about incorporating Yoga and Yoga Nidra into your routine?

Ria: I'm intrigued, especially because they align with some of my interests.

Insomnia Educator: Wonderful. I'll show you some basic poses and meditation practices that are specifically designed to alleviate stress and anxiety.

Ria: Sounds good to me.

Insomnia Educator: Next, let's talk about some Supplementary Aids. We talked about a weighted blanket last time. How do you feel about giving it a try?

Ria: I love the idea, especially since it fits with my room's aesthetic.

Insomnia Educator: Excellent. I'll provide you with some recommendations on where to get one that would suit your needs. Now, how about Natural Aids and Supplements? Have you considered CBD oil?

Ria: I've heard about it, but never really looked into it.

Insomnia Educator: It could be a natural alternative to help you relax. I'll give you some literature on how it might help with sleep.

Ria: I'd like to read that, actually.

Insomnia Educator: Great, let's move on to Environmental Adjustments. We talked about temperature control last time. Any thoughts?

Ria: My room does get a bit warm sometimes, so I'm open to suggestions.

Insomnia Educator: We can discuss some strategies to maintain an optimal sleep environment. Finally, let's talk about Mindful Practices. How do you feel about color journaling with colored pens?

Ria: That sounds really appealing, actually. Like a new form of art therapy for myself.

Insomnia Educator: I thought you might like that! I'll provide you with a journal and some colored pens. We can go through some techniques to help you process your emotions visually before sleep.

Ria: I'm excited to try that!

Insomnia Educator: I'm glad to hear it, Ria! Remember, this is a collaborative endeavor. We'll touch base again in a couple of weeks to see how these strategies are working for you and make any necessary adjustments.

Ria: Sounds like a plan!

With the second conversation, the aim is to sustain the initial trust and rapport built in the first meeting. The focus is on moving Ria towards a more engaged role in her own patient education process.

Helping Ria with Cognitive Distortions

Ria's insomnia is closely tied to her emotional and mental state, fueled by cognitive distortions that amplify her anxieties and stress. These distortions make her already complex situation even more challenging to navigate. The aim is to help her recognize these distorted thought patterns and equip her with tools to challenge them, thereby aiding in the patient education process.

Cognitive Distortions Ria Might Face:
1. **All-or-Nothing Thinking**: Ria may see her art career and personal identity as either a complete success or a total failure, with no middle ground.
2. **Catastrophizing**: She might blow the consequences of her family finding out about her gender identity struggles or her art career not taking off out of proportion.
3. **Should Statements**: Ria may have a list of 'shoulds' and 'should nots' that may be contributing to her anxiety, particularly around family expectations and societal norms.
4. **Personalization and Blame**: She might feel that she's solely responsible for her insomnia or any emotional discomfort within her family.

Conversational Strategies for Addressing Cognitive Distortions:

1. **Socratic Questioning:**
   - "Ria, when you say you're worried about your future in art, what specific thoughts come to mind?"
   - **Reasoning:** This can help her articulate her fears, making it easier to identify any cognitive distortions.

2. **Thought Records:**
   - "Let's jot down instances this week where you felt particularly anxious or couldn't sleep. What were you thinking at that moment?"
   - **Reasoning:** This exercise can make her more aware of her thought patterns, setting the stage for challenging distortions.

3. **Challenging Distortions:**
   - "You mentioned that you feel like a total failure if you don't perfect a piece of art. Is that a fair statement to yourself?"
   - **Reasoning:** Directly challenging a distorted thought can help her see its irrationality.

4. **Positive Reframing:**
   - "Instead of viewing an unfinished art piece as a failure, could it be seen as a work in progress or a learning opportunity?"
   - **Reasoning:** This offers her an alternative, more constructive way to view the situation.

5. **Reality Testing:**
   - "What's the worst that could happen if your art career takes longer to develop, and what steps could you take to handle it?"
   - **Reasoning:** This helps her consider practical steps instead of catastrophizing.

Tools and Exercises:
1. **Thought-Challenging Worksheets**: Provide her with worksheets designed to challenge cognitive distortions.
2. **Mindfulness Techniques**: Introduce mindfulness as a way to become aware of her thoughts without judgment, making it easier to challenge distortions.
3. **Cognitive Restructuring**: Offer her a guided practice to identify, challenge, and change distorted thoughts.

By addressing Ria's cognitive distortions, we not only tackle a significant underlying contributor to her insomnia but also help her navigate her emotional and mental complexities with more clarity. This individualized approach further moves Ria toward a more engaged role in her patient education process

Ria's Progress, Setbacks, and Recovery

Ria delved into her patient education process with mixed feelings—curiosity tinged with caution. Her initial efforts, like the incorporation of Yoga and Yoga Nidra, were steps towards a more balanced emotional state and indirectly enhanced her sleep. The art of color journaling found a special place in her nightly routine, giving her a creative outlet to process complex emotions.

Within the first month, Ria felt a change in the air. The grip of her cognitive distortions loosened a tad, making room for more rational thoughts. Her room, already an aesthetic haven, became a sanctuary, thanks to temperature adjustments that improved her sleep environment. She felt less anxious about her art practice, seeing it less as a battleground of existential questions and more as a space for self-expression.

However, around the third month, Ria confronted some setbacks. Pressures related to her family's matchmaking efforts and her ongoing internal struggle with her gender identity came to a head. This collision of external and internal factors led her to disengage from her newfound practices. Yoga sessions were replaced by restless nights of overthinking, and her color journal lay untouched.

Recognizing this regression, Ria scheduled another session with her insomnia educator. The conversation focused on examining the triggers for her recent setbacks and the cognitive distortions that had resurfaced. Ria then transitioned to "worry journaling." By jotting down her anxieties and symbolically closing the book, Ria felt a sense of relief, giving her permission to set aside those concerns, even if only for the night.

During this recovery phase, Ria was introduced to the concept of self-compassion. The educator reminded her that setbacks are natural and that showing kindness to oneself is crucial in these moments. This principle resonated with Ria's artistic sensibilities, adding another layer to her emotional resilience toolkit.

The following period of Ria's sleep education journey told a story of resilience. Despite the ups and downs, the prevailing theme remained one of self-awareness and creative adaptability. Not only did Ria manage to navigate the complexities of insomnia, but she also found a renewed sense of self in the process.

Ria's story serves as a testament to the complexities of the patient education process, especially when intersecting with diverse emotional and social landscapes. It speaks to the enduring human spirit, showing that setbacks are not failures but rather opportunities for growth and adaptation.

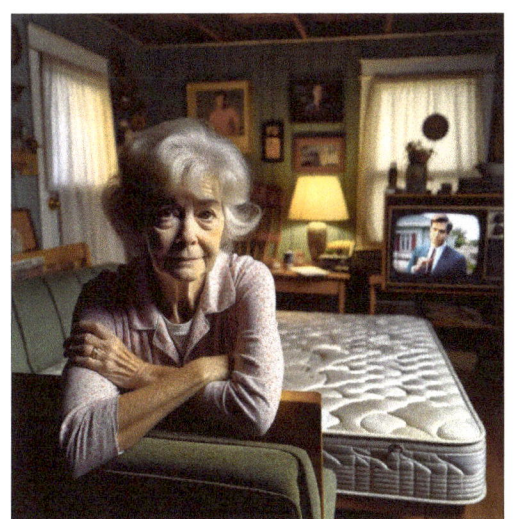

The Restless Retiree

Hannah, a 66-year-old retiree, lives alone in a cozy apartment in Nashville, TN. Full of sweetness and highly motivated, she loves to talk and share stories. She spent 40 years as a legal secretary, where her meticulousness was highly valued. She's a devout volunteer at her local church, always the first to offer a helping hand for community events or bake sales.

Hannah has chronic back pain, which led her to misuse opioid painkillers for a period. She managed to discontinue the opioids with the help of a strict pain management program but now struggles with lingering insomnia. Her symptoms include difficulty falling asleep, frequent wake-ups during the night, and trouble falling back asleep. These issues are exacerbated by her chronic back pain and an old, uncomfortable mattress that is over 25 years old, making restful sleep elusive.

Hannah's apartment can get cluttered, but she finds that keeping it neat makes her feel more relaxed. She loves watching Perry Mason reruns and finds that they have a soporific effect when they air in the afternoon, although this doesn't help her maintain a full night's sleep. She wishes she could exercise more, particularly to TV exercise programs she enjoys, but her cramped living space makes it challenging.

Highly motivated to improve her situation, Hannah was referred by her sleep physician to an insomnia patient educator. She's very open to learning and is eager for "real, practical solutions" to improve her sleep. Her Intrinsic Motivation Inventory (IMI) scores are quite high, indicating a strong willingness to make lifestyle changes to improve her sleep quality.

Having the Clinical Conversation with Hannah

Setting: A cozy, well-lit consultation room within a sleep medicine practice. The room features medical literature about sleep disorders. Hannah sits across from the insomnia educator, her eyes bright and engaged but her demeanor slightly reserved.

1. **"Hannah, you've dealt with chronic back pain for quite some time, and more recently, you've been experiencing insomnia. How has that been affecting your daily life lately?"**
   - **Reasoning**: This opens up the conversation about her chronic conditions and invites her to share her experiences.
2. **"Family is important to you, but it seems like discussions around health can get a bit tense. Could you expand on that a little?"**
- **Reasoning**: Acknowledging the importance of family in her life while gently probing into an area of tension allows for a deeper understanding of her social support network.

3. **"I noticed you have a soft spot for antique teacups. How does collecting them bring joy to your life?"**
   - **Reasoning**: Switching to a lighter topic that she's passionate about can make the conversation more engaging and provide insight into her coping mechanisms.
4. **"You mentioned a recent fall that you think was due to sleep issues. Could you tell me more about how that event influenced your decision to get professional help?"**
   - **Reasoning**: This focuses on a key event that spurred action, providing insights into her perceptions and readiness to change.
5. **"Your Intrinsic Motivation Inventory scores are quite high, which is encouraging. How willing are you to make some changes to improve your sleep?"**
   - **Reasoning**: Discussing her IMI scores gives a sense of her motivation level and opens the door to conversations about potential interventions.
6. **"You've said you're looking for real, practical solutions and aren't a fan of what some might call 'fringe' treatments. Could you help me understand what you consider to be practical?"**
   - **Reasoning**: This question directly addresses her skepticism and sets the stage for aligning the patient education process with her expectations and comfort zone.
7. **"You seem to enjoy courtroom dramas and crosswords. Ever notice if these activities have any impact—good or bad—on your sleep?"**
   - **Reasoning**: This leads into a discussion about lifestyle factors affecting her sleep and helps in tailoring recommendations.

Building Hannah's Education Plan

With Hannah's high levels of motivation and her preference for straightforward, practical solutions, the educator has both an opportunity and a challenge: to leverage her willingness to engage while navigating her specific needs and skepticism.

Hannah's insomnia manifests as a complex interplay between her chronic back pain, past misuse of opioid painkillers, and a change in sleep architecture that often accompanies aging. Her high IMI scores indicate a strong willingness to improve her sleep, offering an excellent starting point for evidence-based interventions.

Traditional Eastern Remedies:

Acupressure:
- **Recommendation**: Introduce the idea of acupressure as a non-invasive method to manage back pain.
- **Teaching Method**: Review a few handouts on acupressure techniques she can self-administer.

Mindful Practices:

Progressive Muscle Relaxation:
- **Recommendation**: Given her back pain, this technique could help in relaxing her muscles before sleep.
- **Teaching Method**: Guide her through a live session to show her how to tense and relax muscle groups.

Lifestyle Hacks:

Grandchild Assisted Home Organization:
- **Recommendation**: Arrange for one of her grandchildren to visit once a month to help clean and organize her apartment, as a tidy environment helps her relax before sleep.
- **Teaching Method**: Discuss the benefits of maintaining an organized living space and its positive effects on sleep. Additionally, create a simple monthly checklist to guide the organizing session with her grandchild.

Perry Mason Pre-Sleep Routine:
- **Recommendation**: Incorporate watching Perry Mason into her pre-sleep routine, as it has a tendency to make her feel sleepy.
- **Teaching Method**: Discuss the idea of using television shows as a cue for sleep readiness. Encourage her to pay attention to how she feels as she watches and to turn off the TV and attempt sleep as soon as she starts to feel drowsy.

Natural Aids and Supplements:

Herbal Teas:
- **Recommendation**: Explore teas like chamomile or valerian root as part of a pre-sleep ritual.
- **Teaching Method**: Conduct a tea-tasting session during one of the consultations.

Environmental Adjustments:

Mattress Replacement:
- **Recommendation**: Given her 25-year-old mattress, it's time for an upgrade.
- **Teaching Method**: Discuss the types of mattresses that could help alleviate her back pain.

The Second Clinical Conversation with Hannah

Setting: *A well-lit room in a local medical center specializing in sleep medicine. The room is adorned with informative medical literature on sleep disorders, and a charming tea set featuring antique teacups is displayed on a side table. Patient Educator greets Hannah with a warm smile as she takes her seat, visibly motivated but also a bit curious about what's to come.*

Patient Educator: Hannah, it's great to see you again. How have you been feeling since our last meeting?

Hannah: I've been eager to see what you've put together for me!

Patient Educator: Wonderful! Let's start with some Traditional Eastern Remedies. Have you ever considered acupressure for your chronic back pain?

Hannah: Acupressure? I'm not familiar with it.

Patient Educator: It's a non-invasive technique that could help you manage your back pain. I can show you some basic techniques you can do at home.

Hannah: That sounds interesting, I'm willing to try.

Patient Educator: Excellent. Next on the list is Mindful Practices. How do you feel about progressive muscle relaxation?

Hannah: I'm not sure what that is, but I'm open to learning!

Patient Educator: It's a technique that involves tensing and relaxing your muscles. It could help you wind down before sleep, especially given your back issues.

Hannah: Anything to help my back and my sleep is worth trying!

Patient Educator: I'm pleased to hear that! Now, let's talk about some Lifestyle Hacks. One idea is to invite one of your grandchildren over once a month to help you clean and organize your apartment. What do you think?

Hannah: Oh, that's a fabulous idea! A clean home always makes me feel more relaxed.

Patient Educator: Perfect! And since you find Perry Mason so sleep-inducing, how about making it a part of your pre-sleep routine?

Hannah: I never thought about it, but it does make sense!

Patient Educator: Great! Moving on to Natural Aids and Supplements, how about incorporating some herbal teas like chamomile or valerian root before bed?

Hannah: I do enjoy a good cup of tea.

Patient Educator: Lastly, let's discuss Environmental Adjustments. You've had your mattress for quite a long time, and a new one could make a world of difference for your back pain and sleep quality.

Hannah: You're probably right. It's been more than two decades, after all.

Patient Educator: We can go over some options that would be suitable for you, focusing on those that could help alleviate your back pain.

Hannah: I appreciate that. It's a lot to take in, but I'm excited to start making these changes.

Patient Educator: That's the spirit, Hannah! Remember, this is a collaborative effort. After two weeks, we'll meet again to see how things are going and make any necessary adjustments.

Hannah: I'm looking forward to it!

Helping Hannah with Cognitive Distortions

Navigating the intricate web of insomnia is not just about implementing lifestyle hacks or making environmental adjustments. It's also crucial to tackle the cognitive distortions that might be amplifying Hannah's sleep difficulties. Given her strong-willed nature, it's quite possible that these thought patterns are deeply ingrained and thus contribute to her insomnia. By identifying these distortions and offering strategies for cognitive restructuring, we can give Hannah the tools she needs to challenge these automatic negative thoughts. This is an essential step in breaking the cycle of sleepless nights and the daytime distress they cause.

Polarized Thinking About Health
- **Distortion**: "If I can't get a full night of sleep, then the entire day is ruined."
- **Cognitive Restructuring**: "Even a few hours of quality sleep can be beneficial and doesn't mean the day is a total loss. Let's focus on incremental improvements."

Overgeneralization Regarding Medical Guidance
- **Distortion**: "Doctors never have practical solutions; they're all the same."
- **Cognitive Restructuring**: "Each healthcare provider is different, and some may offer advice or treatments that can genuinely help me. I should remain open to different perspectives."

Catastrophizing the Impact of Sleeplessness
- **Distortion**: "If I can't fix my sleep problems, my health will deteriorate completely."
- **Cognitive Restructuring**: "While sleep is crucial for health, it's just one of many factors. There are strategies I can employ to manage sleep issues and improve overall well-being."

Labeling Self Due to Chronic Pain
- **Distortion**: "I must be weak to let this back pain affect me so much."
- **Cognitive Restructuring**: "Chronic pain is a medical condition, not a sign of personal weakness. It's okay to seek help and manage it effectively."

Personalization in Family Interactions
- **Distortion**: "My children don't listen to me about my health because they don't care."
- **Cognitive Restructuring**: "They might be frustrated or unsure how to help. Their actions are not necessarily a reflection of their love or concern for me."

Mental Filtering When Considering Sleep Aids
- **Distortion**: "Herbal teas and other natural aids are all just nonsense. If they can't fix my sleep, nothing can."
- **Cognitive Restructuring**: "Different approaches work for different people. Just because one method doesn't work doesn't mean another won't. I should consider a broad spectrum of evidence-based options."

Should Statements Regarding Sleep
- **Distortion**: "I should be able to fall asleep as soon as I lie down."
- **Cognitive Restructuring**: "Sleep is a complex process influenced by many factors, including stress and environment. It's not about 'should'; it's about finding what works for me."

Through targeted cognitive restructuring, Hannah can learn to challenge these distortions, providing her with a more balanced and constructive perspective. This mental shift is crucial for alleviating her insomnia symptoms and improving her overall quality of life.

Hannah's Progress, Setbacks & Recovery

Hannah started her journey with an unquenchable thirst for improvement. She was proactive in implementing the recommendations made during her patient education sessions. Acupressure became a daily ritual, progressively easing her back pain and indirectly improving her sleep quality. The monthly visits from her grandchildren turned into mini home-makeover sessions, leaving her apartment tidier and her mind more tranquil.

Her pre-sleep routine now included an episode of Perry Mason, a cue that helped signal to her body that it was time to wind down. Even her skepticism toward herbal teas waned as she found that a cup of chamomile before bed actually did help her relax.

Within the first month, Hannah was thrilled with the progress. Her sleep had improved noticeably, the number of wake-ups had decreased, and she even found herself falling asleep faster. She felt more energetic for her volunteer activities and less anxious overall.

However, life has a way of throwing curveballs. Around the six-month mark, Hannah faced an emotional setback when a close friend passed away. The grief and the responsibilities of helping to organize community memorial events took a toll on her, both emotionally and physically.

Caught in the whirlwind of emotions and responsibilities, she neglected her newfound insomnia remedies. Episodes of Perry Mason were replaced by late-night phone calls with friends who were also grieving. The loss disrupted her sleep routine, leading her to revert to her old cognitive distortions. She found herself thinking, "If I can't sleep because of this emotional turmoil, my health will just keep deteriorating."

Recognizing that she had relapsed into her previous sleep-disrupting habits, Hannah reached out to her to a grief and loss therapist who helped her understand the power of self-compassion. "Your feelings are natural given the circumstances, Hannah," said counselor. "But remember, your sleep and health are also important. Let's revisit some strategies that you might have overlooked during this challenging time."

The educator emphasized the importance of compartmentalizing her worries, particularly when it came to the emotional stresses tied to her friend's passing. She was introduced to "worry journaling," similar to what helped Janice. By writing down her concerns and closing the book, Hannah found she could symbolically put those worries to rest for the night.

Self-compassion became a cornerstone in her recovery. During this period, the patient educator emphasized the importance of kindness towards oneself, especially when things don't go as planned. This aligned with Hannah's community-centered values, adding another layer to her resilience toolkit.

The subsequent period of Hannah's journey told a tale of resurgence. Despite the inevitable bumps on the road, the prevailing narrative was one of self-discovery and empowerment. Hannah not only regained her sleep equilibrium but also reaffirmed her commitment to living her retired years to the fullest, chronic back pain and all.

Thus, Hannah's story is one that portrays the ebb and flow of the patient education process. It's a testament to the value of adaptability and the enduring human spirit, showing that setbacks are but stepping stones on the path to better sleep and, by extension, a better life.

Joe, The Sleep-Seeking Soldier

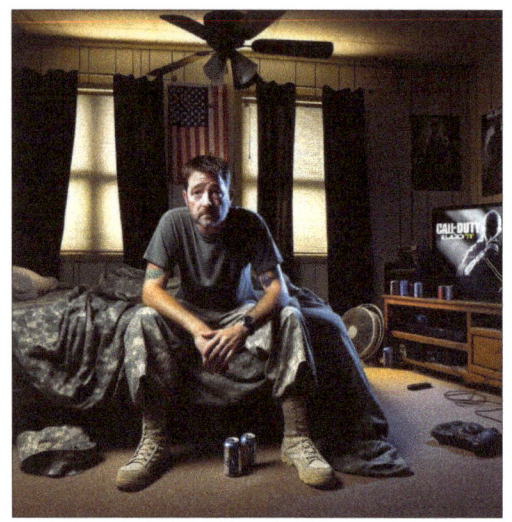

In the heart of San Antonio, Texas, Joe, an Iraq War veteran, is ensnared in a battle between his storied past and his present struggles. His austere apartment, a stone's throw from Fort Sam Houston, stands as a bastion against the disorder outside. Blackout curtains shield against both sunlight and haunting recollections, while a ceiling fan's constant motion evokes memories of his service.

Nightly, Joe confronts the dread of sleep as a gateway to his nightmares, a time when his vigilant mind resists the surrender to troubling dreams. Seeking distraction, he turns to video games like Call of Duty, which ironically amplify the restlessness they're meant to mitigate.

The chasm between Joe and his girlfriend, Emma—a spirited lover of the outdoors and vibrant murals that color the city's parks—grows with each passing day. Their conversations, once filled with plans for hikes and picnics, now often dissolve into arguments, leaving a residue of frustration and confusion. Emma tries to understand, to connect with Joe on a level that transcends the barriers he's erected, but it's like reaching for a mirage.

Sharing a bed has become an ordeal. Joe's hyper-alertness to every shift and sigh from Emma is a reflex that rips him from the fragile grip of sleep. Every unintentional nudge is a potential threat, sparking a rush of adrenaline that shatters any hope of tranquility.

Joe's intellect, a sharp tool honed by a natural curiosity for science and the mechanics of the world around him, offers little solace in the shadowy hours of the night. Evenings bring its own ritual—many cans of beer have been a misguided salve for his frayed nerves. Joe clings to the belief that booze helps usher in sleep, but each sip only leads to more fragmented rest, leaving him more depleted with the morning.

In his youth, Joe was a deep sleeper and had few problems settling down for the night. Now, after his military service, he's driven to a point of desperation and seeks the expertise of a physician to alleviate his insomnia. While the temporary medication prescribed offers a fleeting reprieve, aiding him in his quest for sleep, Joe remains aware that this remedy is not a lasting solution.

Having the Clinical Conversation with Joe

Setting: *In a quiet, private room tucked within the bright corridors of a bustling primary care physician's group, the hum of the city fades into a distant murmur. The space is furnished with comfort in mind—a round table anchors the room, flanked by ergonomic chairs that promise a reprieve from the day's weariness. Here, Joe sits, his posture a mix of a soldier's alertness and a weary traveler's slump, across from the patient educator, a beacon of guidance amid his tumultuous quest for rest. The session begins with a nod of mutual respect and an empathetic smile.*

Questions:
1. "Joe, as you settle into the evening, what are some thoughts or routines that you notice becoming more prominent?"
2. "Reflecting on your nightly routine, could you walk me through how you prepare for bed and if there's anything in particular that you find comforting or unsettling?"
3. "You've shared that gaming has been both a refuge and a source of tension for you. Can you explore that dichotomy a bit more with me?"
4. "Emma has been a significant part of your life. In what ways does your relationship with her intersect with your sleep experiences?"
5. "You've mentioned your natural curiosity and interest in science. How does this aspect of your personality play into your understanding or approach to your sleep challenges?"

6. In a gentle shift towards motivational interviewing, the educator leans in slightly, "Joe, on a scale from 1 to 10, how ready do you feel to make changes that could potentially improve your sleep, and what do you think it would take to move you just one point higher on that scale?"

These questions aim to open up a dialogue that gives Joe the space to explore his experiences and feelings related to his insomnia, without making assumptions about his condition or pushing him toward specific responses. The motivational interviewing question is particularly aimed at gauging Joe's readiness to change and to understand his perspective on the importance of addressing his sleep issues.

Building Joe's Education Plan

Joe's insomnia is a multifaceted challenge, deeply rooted in his military history and compounded by his lifestyle and psychological state. His unique situation requires a blend of traditional and modern approaches, digital solutions, and environmental adjustments, all tailored to his individual needs and interests.

Possible Recommendations for Joe's Insomnia Education Plan

Lifestyle Hacks:

Routine Establishment:

- **Recommendation:** Transition to calming video games like "The Elder Scrolls V: Skyrim" or "Divinity: Original Sin 2" two hours before bed to engage Joe's mind without overstimulating it.
- **Teaching Method:** Compare the strategic planning and immersive worlds of Role Playing Games (RPGs) to military strategy and scientific exploration, showing how they can be both engaging and conducive to winding down.

Digital Age Solutions:

Sleep Tracking:

- **Recommendation:** Utilize the "Sleep Cycle" app or similar, to record sleep patterns and nocturnal sounds, providing Joe with evidence that his environment remains secure throughout the night.
- **Teaching Method:** Demonstrate the app's functionality and discuss how it can integrate into his nightly routine, serving as both a scientific interest and a reassurance tool.

Environmental Adjustments:

Bedroom Modifications:

- **Recommendation:** Remove the ceiling fan that triggers military barracks memories and replace it with a stationary air purifier or a quiet standing fan to maintain airflow without the visual disturbance.
- **Teaching Method:** Explain the psychological benefits of altering environmental triggers and how this can create a more peaceful and restful bedroom space.

Natural Light Engagement:

- **Recommendation:** Encourage Joe to spend 10 minutes in the early morning and at sunset in natural light to help regulate his sleep-wake cycle.
- **Teaching Method:** Use scientific explanations to describe how light exposure affects melatonin production and the body's circadian rhythms, potentially delving into the role of adenosine as a 'sleep pressure' chemical.
    - ADENOSINE: Engaging with natural light during early morning and at sunset can indeed play a part in sleep readiness. Exposure to natural light in the morning helps reset the circadian rhythm, promoting alertness and reducing melatonin production, the hormone that makes you feel sleepy. Conversely, the dimming light at sunset signals the brain to increase melatonin production, preparing the body for sleep. Adenosine, on the

other hand, gradually accumulates in the brain during wakefulness, promoting the drive to sleep. While light exposure and adenosine both contribute to sleep regulation, they function through different mechanisms within the sleep-wake cycle.

Clinical and Therapeutic Methods:

PTSD Management:
- **Recommendation:** Provide a PTSD referral sheet for specialized therapy that can assist with relationship and occupational challenges.
- **Teaching Method:** Outline the benefits of targeted PTSD therapy, emphasizing how managing PTSD symptoms can significantly improve sleep quality and relationship dynamics.

Alcohol Consumption:
- **Recommendation:** Encourage Joe to become more aware of his alcohol consumption patterns, particularly in relation to his sleep quality. Rather than aiming for reduction, the goal is for Joe to track his intake for two weeks and gradually delay his last drink of the night, moving the time back by one hour increments until he stops drinking about four hours before bedtime.
- **Teaching Method:** Provide Joe with a simple tracking sheet for his alcohol intake, along with a handout that explains how alcohol can affect sleep. This educational material should detail the stages of sleep and how alcohol can disrupt the sleep cycle, emphasizing the importance of the timing of alcohol consumption relative to bedtime.
- This approach respects Joe's autonomy and provides him with the tools to make informed decisions about his drinking habits in relation to his sleep health. It's a non-confrontational method that facilitates self-awareness and self-regulation, which can be empowering for Joe as he navigates his path to better sleep.

- **Recommendation:** Implement a gradual reduction in alcohol use, with a focus on tracking and understanding its impact on sleep.
- **Teaching Method:** Offer Joe a structured tracking system and educational materials that illustrate the relationship between alcohol consumption and sleep architecture.

To resonate with Joe's structured military background and his scientific intellect, the plan should be presented in a clear, sequential, and evidence-based manner. Here's how we can structure the presentation:

- **Structured Guide:** Offer a detailed, step-by-step guide for implementing each aspect of the plan, employing military and scientific terminology for familiarity and engagement.
- **Visual Aids:** Create charts and infographics that clearly show how Joe's new routine can lead to improved sleep, appealing to his analytical mind.
- **Audiovisual Materials:** Provide audio recordings for mindfulness and relaxation exercises, as well as podcasts that align with his interests, for use in his pre-sleep routine.
- **Personalized Feedback:** Set up a system for Joe to receive feedback based on his app data and sleep diary, ensuring the plan remains responsive to his needs and progress.

The plan's presentation should resonate with Joe's logical and disciplined nature, providing him with a sense of control and engagement in his journey toward better sleep. Each recommendation should reinforce the idea that small, incremental changes can lead to significant improvements in his sleep quality and overall well-being.

The Second Clinical Conversation with Joe

Setting: A sleep medicine practice office space, radiating a sense of calm professionalism. The room is equipped with a large screen prepared for a presentation, signaling a transition *from exploratory discussion to action planning. The patient educator offers Joe a warm yet confident smile, an unspoken message of readiness to embark on the next phase of his journey towards better sleep.*

Patient Educator: "Joe, it's good to have you back. After our initial conversation, I've put together a plan that's specifically designed with your experiences and lifestyle in mind. Are you ready to go through it together?"

Joe: "Yes, I've been looking forward to this."

Patient Educator: "Great. We'll start with Lifestyle Hacks. You've mentioned your evening routine includes playing *Call of Duty*. I suggest transitioning to games like 'The Elder Scrolls V: Skyrim' or 'Divinity: Original Sin 2' around two hours before bed. They offer rich stories, combat strategies without the quick reflex twitch-type intensity of first-person shooters. What are your thoughts?"

Joe: "I'm open to it. Those games sound interesting, and if they help, why not?"

Patient Educator: "Excellent. Now, regarding your sleep environment, I believe replacing the ceiling fan that reminds you of the barracks might help. Perhaps a stationary air purifier for airflow without movement could be a comforting alternative."

Joe: "That makes sense. I hadn't thought about the fan that way, but I'm willing to try changing it."

Patient Educator: "Moving on to Digital Age Solutions, let's utilize a sleep tracker like 'Sleep Cycle.' It records sleep patterns and nighttime sounds, which could provide reassurance that your environment is secure while you sleep."

Joe: "I'm a bit of a data guy, so seeing the stats might actually be good for me."

Patient Educator: "I thought you might appreciate that approach. Now, concerning alcohol, let's focus on mindfulness. Track your consumption for awareness without immediately aiming for reduction. Just note the times you drink and gradually delay the last drink each night by an hour until you're about four hours clear before bed."

Joe: "So, no pressure to cut back drastically, just track and adjust slowly?"

Patient Educator: "Precisely. It's all about informed decisions. Lastly, let's touch on the PTSD symptoms you've worked on over the years. Here's a referral sheet of clinical providers who can provide specialized therapy for managing PTSD symptoms, which can significantly impact sleep quality."

Joe: "I'll have a look. Even though I've been to therapy in the past, I know that's an area I have to stay on top of if I want things to get better."

Patient Educator: "With your dedication, I have no doubt it will be, Joe. Let's schedule a check-in sometime in the next few weeks."

The session concludes with a sense of shared commitment, the educator confident in Joe's potential for progress, and Joe armed with a personalized plan to tackle his sleep challenges.

Helping Joe with Cognitive Distortions

Addressing Joe's insomnia involves not only lifestyle changes and environmental modifications but also confronting cognitive distortions that exacerbate his sleep challenges. As a soldier dealing with PTSD, Joe's cognitive distortions are intertwined with his experiences and affect his ability to find restful sleep. Below we outline these distortions and propose cognitive restructuring strategies.

1. **Catastrophizing Military Experiences:**
   - Distortion: "If I let down my guard and have a nightmare, it means I'm back to square one with my PTSD."
   - Cognitive Restructuring: "Nightmares are a common reaction to PTSD and not an indicator of failure. Each day is a step in my ongoing journey of healing."

2. **Hyper-Vigilance During Nighttime:**
   - Distortion: "The moment I close my eyes, I'm vulnerable to unseen dangers."
   - Cognitive Restructuring: "I've created a safe haven in my home, and it's okay to embrace rest. Being vigilant is a part of my past, not a requirement for my present."

3. **Overgeneralization of Threats:**
   - Distortion: "Every unexpected sound could be an imminent threat, just like in war."
   - Cognitive Restructuring: "Sounds in my environment are normal urban life, not the battlefield. It's safe to acknowledge them without alarm."

4. **Emotional Reasoning in Response to Triggers:**
   - Distortion: "When I feel scared, it's because danger is real."
   - Cognitive Restructuring: "My feelings are powerful but not always indicative of current reality. Recognizing this can help me navigate false alarms."

5. **Personalization of Sleep Struggles:**
   - Distortion: "I should be able to control my sleep; failing to do so is a weakness."
   - Cognitive Restructuring: "Sleep difficulties are a common response to trauma. It's not about control but about learning new strategies for rest."

6. **Selective Abstraction on Setbacks:**
   - Distortion: "A bad night of sleep is evidence that my strategies aren't effective."
   - Cognitive Restructuring: "Healing isn't linear. I'll look at patterns over time rather than isolated incidents."

7. **Mental Filtering:**
   - Distortion: "I had a week of better sleep, but one bad night makes me feel it was all for nothing."
   - Cognitive Restructuring: "I will have good nights and challenging nights. Each night is a new opportunity for rest, not a verdict on my progress."

Joe's Progress, Setbacks, and Recovery

Joe embarked on the patient education process with a mix of hope and inherent caution, fully aware of his need for change yet conscious of his past's enduring hold on his nights. He noticed improvements as he adopted the new strategies: engaging with less stimulating video games in the evenings began to smooth his transition to sleep, and removing the ceiling fan from his bedroom reduced the sensory echoes of his military service. Joe delved into the science of adenosine's impact on sleep and shared his findings with Emma. They committed to spending time in the early morning and evening light, hoping to leverage the science of light exposure to improve his sleep-wake cycle.

Despite these steps forward, Joe faced setbacks. The anniversary of a harrowing military event, in which he lost a fellow soldier, triggered a resurgence of nightmares and sleep disruption. In response, Joe reverted to alcohol, his longstanding but maladaptive coping mechanism. Rather than seeing this as a backslide, Joe reached out for help, engaging in talk therapy bi-weekly, a resource he discovered through a brochure provided by his patient educator.

In therapy, Joe and his counselor worked on cognitive restructuring strategies, centering on his resilience and capacity for recovery. They introduced the concept of "Continued

Courage in Recovery," reinforcing the idea that healing is a non-linear journey marked by persistence and adaptability, not a quest for perfection.

In the weeks that followed, Joe earnestly tried to realign with his plan, adapting it to better fit the reality of his experiences. He embraced a more flexible approach, learning to navigate the ebb and flow of progress without harsh self-judgment.

Joe's story, however, took a turn that underscores the unpredictable and challenging nature of insomnia, particularly when intertwined with PTSD and substance abuse. Despite his understanding of the importance of controlling his sleep and his earnest efforts, he remained ensnared by the cognitive distortion that equated difficulty sleeping with personal failure. This belief, unyielding and harsh, drove him to escalate his drinking, leading to blackouts. One night, lost in an alcoholic blackout, he found himself in an altercation and, in a subsequent fit of rage, attempted to drive home—only to be arrested for DUI. Emma, strained by his refusal to seek employment and stop drinking, parted ways with him. The last known chapter of Joe's story was a somber one: he had not completed the alcohol abuse treatment at the VA clinic and was last known to be living on the streets.

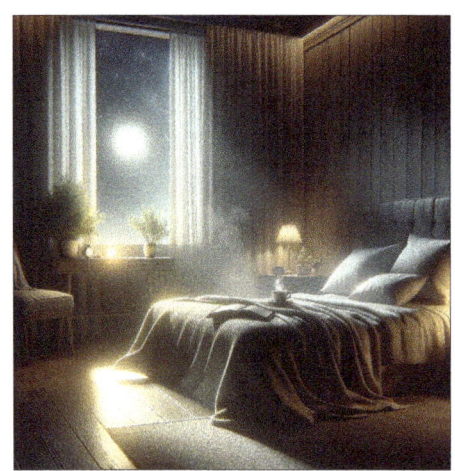

Note on Insomnia Recovery

Joe's experience is a poignant reminder that the journey through insomnia, especially when compounded by other mental health challenges, is fraught with unpredictability. Recovery is not a guarantee, and interventions do not work uniformly for everyone. The intricacies of each individual's experience with insomnia make it a particularly challenging condition to treat. Joe's case illustrates that even with the right tools and support, the road to recovery can take unexpected turns. It's crucial to recognize that setbacks are not simply obstacles; they are part of the complex human experience. Understanding and acknowledging this can foster more compassionate and realistic approaches to managing insomnia and its related conditions.

Epilogue–
The Illusion of Sleep Health:
When Good Enough Sleep is Good Enough

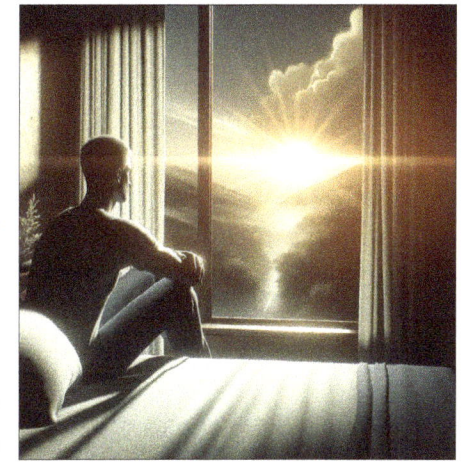

At the heart of our understanding of sleep health lies a simple, yet profound question posed by sleep physician, Jonathan Warren, MD, ABSM: "Do I feel rested?" This question encapsulates the essence of sleep health, transcending the myriad of remedies and approaches to insomnia. It's a reminder that, despite the complexity of sleep science and social judgments, the ultimate goal is to achieve a state of restfulness that resonates on a personal level.

So, this question "Do I feel rested?" challenges us to look beyond traditional sleep metrics, focusing instead on the individual's subjective experience of restfulness. This approach aligns with the emerging sociocultural perspectives on sleep, which recognize its multifaceted nature and the diverse factors influencing it. By redefining what it means to be truly rested, we open the door to a more personalized and empathetic approach in our client education process, one that respects the unique sleep experiences and needs of each individual.

The Commodification of Sleep

In recent years, sleep has transcended into a significant economic and sociocultural phenomenon. This transformation is evident in the burgeoning sleep industry, which capitalizes on the universal quest for better sleep. According to a report by McKinsey & Company, the sleep-health industry was valued at approximately $30 to $40 billion as of 2017, with a growth rate of more than 8% annually. This rapid expansion reflects a growing public obsession with achieving optimal sleep.

Megan Garber's insights in "The Protestant Sleep Ethic" illuminate how sleep has become a status symbol in modern society. The narrative surrounding sleep now often includes a moral dimension, where the quantity and quality of one's sleep are seen as reflections of personal virtue or success. This perspective is further complicated by figures like Elon Musk, who publicly glorify sleep deprivation, inadvertently promoting a culture where rest is undervalued. While Musk has been known for his statements that seemingly undervalue rest, it's important to consider the broader picture of Musk's ilk. Employees at Musk's companies have noted that the portrayal of relentless work with little sleep is more of a myth than a constant reality. They acknowledge that while there are intense periods of work, known as "sprints," and urgent situations that require immediate attention, but the idea of consistently curled up in a sleeping bag under one's desk is not a standard practice.

In a 2023 podcast with AI Scientist, Lex Fridman, Musk himself addressed this topic, offering a personal insight into his own sleep habits saying that he needs at least six hours of sleep per night to function effectively, that his performance significantly deteriorates with inadequate sleep. This admission from Musk is critical, as it challenges the one-dimensional portrayal of high-achieving individuals neglecting sleep for success.

Sleep Inequality: Socioeconomic and Geopolitical Factors

The financial aspect of sleep solutions has widened the gap in sleep health. High-quality sleep aids and technologies are often expensive, making them inaccessible to lower-income individuals. This disparity leads to a troubling scenario where quality sleep becomes a luxury rather than a basic right, exacerbating issues of sleep inequality.

Sleep, often perceived as a universal human experience, is significantly influenced by socioeconomic and geopolitical factors. The disparities in sleep quality and access to sleep health resources between different social strata and in varying global contexts are profound and warrant close examination.

Individuals in lower socioeconomic classes often face numerous challenges that adversely affect their sleep. Factors such as financial stress, job insecurity, substandard living conditions, and environmental noise contribute to poor sleep quality. These conditions can lead to a range of sleep disorders, from insomnia to sleep apnea, often going undiagnosed and untreated due to limited access to healthcare resources. The cumulative effect of these stressors disrupts the natural sleep cycle, leading to chronic sleep deprivation and its associated health risks.

In war-torn regions, the situation is even more dire. The constant stress and trauma associated with living in conflict zones severely disrupt sleep patterns. Frequent exposure to violence, displacement, and the loss of loved ones create a state of hyperarousal and anxiety, making restful sleep nearly impossible. Children and adults in these environments often suffer from persistent nightmares and insomnia, exacerbating the mental and physical toll of the conflict.

In Daniel J. Buysse's article "Sleep Health: Can We Define It? Does It Matter?", the importance of defining sleep health is underscored. Defining sleep health with quantifiable degrees within the normal range and concrete targets for health promotion aligns with broader agendas like improving population health and identifying biomarkers efficiently. The good working definition of sleep health, according to Buysse is as follows: "Sleep health is a multidimensional pattern of sleep-wakefulness, adapted to individual, social, and environmental demands, promoting physical and mental well-being. Good sleep health is characterized by subjective satisfaction, appropriate timing, adequate duration, high efficiency, and sustained alertness during waking hours."

This definition highlights that sleep health is not specific to any sleep disorder but focuses on measurable attributes in individuals, adaptable across different situations and age groups. However, this definition should emphasis balanced judgment ensuring that effective sleep health strategies are accessible to all, not just those who can afford them.

The Morality of Sleep

The moral judgments surrounding sleep in American culture, brilliantly explored not only by Megan Garber, but by Jenna Ryu, in a 2023 piece on a trending term "bed rotting," the concept of spending extended periods in bed engaging in leisurely activities, often as a form of self-care, challenging the judgment that bed-rotting is just laziness. They reflect this resting landscape with ethical implications. Not only does there seem to be a class divide in sleep, highlighted by Silicon Valley's glorification of sleep sacrifice, but Garber points out that "we as a culture tend to only praise certain types of self-care—you know, the socially acceptable one like attending a workout class or listen to an enlightening podcast." One is not supposed to waste time binge watching a show on Netflix in our hustle culture.

Jenna Ryu dismantles narrow-minded views of sleep and rest, allowing for a more inclusive understanding that respects individual differences, exclaiming, "Bed rotting can be a very legit form of self-care. It's called rest, people!"

Bravo.

Reevaluating Screen Time Restrictions And Adapting to Modern Realities

In the ever-evolving digital landscape of the 21st century, the concept of a complete screen-time shutdown before bedtime is facing scrutiny. While conventional wisdom has long advocated for disconnecting from screens to ensure a good night's sleep, modern lifestyles and technological advancements have prompted a reevaluation of this practice.

- **The Role of Screens:** Screens have become an integral part of our daily routines. Smartphones serve as alarm clocks, meditation tools, and relaxation companions. The accessibility of soothing apps, calming music, and sleep-inducing content on these devices has redefined how we prepare for sleep.
- **Blue Light Blocking:** With the rise of awareness about the potential sleep-disrupting effects of blue light emitted by screens, many individuals have turned to blue light blocking glasses and screen filters. These technologies enable us to continue using screens while minimizing the potential negative impact on our sleep-wake cycle.
- **Personalized Content:** It's no secret that the type of content we consume before bed can greatly affect our sleep quality. While binge-watching thrilling shows or engaging in intense gaming might not be conducive to sleep,

selectively choosing calming and comforting content on platforms like YouTube or streaming services can actually help us wind down.
- **Flexibility and Adaptation:** The key lies in adapting screen usage to our individual needs and preferences. For some, watching a short, relaxing video or listening to a guided meditation on a mobile device can serve as a pre-sleep ritual, helping them unwind and prepare mentally for rest. Restricting screen time entirely may be unnecessarily restrictive for those who have found a healthy balance.

Personalizing Insomnia Management: Beyond Standardized Fixes

While behavioral methods like relaxation therapy, sleep restriction, and stimulus control therapy recommend getting out of bed when unable to sleep, it's important to recognize that this approach might not be suitable for everyone. Some individuals may not find it necessary to leave the bed to reduce frustration associated with insomnia. Here's why:

Individual Variability: Not all individuals experience the same level of frustration when unable to sleep. For some, simply staying in bed and engaging in a calming activity like reading a book or practicing relaxation exercises may be sufficient to reduce frustration and promote sleep onset without the need to get up.
- Sarah, a 32-year-old graphic designer, experiences occasional insomnia due to work-related stress. She finds that staying in bed and engaging in her art journal, sketching, or painting when she can't sleep reduces her frustration and often leads to a calm state, facilitating sleep onset.

Comfort and Safety: For certain individuals, getting out of bed in the middle of the night may not be comfortable or safe. This could be due to physical limitations, age, or environmental factors. Encouraging them to remain in bed and practice relaxation techniques may be more appropriate in these cases.
- John, a 68-year-old retiree, has been coping with chronic insomnia for many years. His age and the layout of his two-story house with steep stairs make it unsafe for

him to get out of bed at night. Instead, he listens to classical music on a small radio by his bedside, which helps him relax and eventually fall asleep safely.

Sleep Associations: While the primary goal of getting out of bed is to disassociate the bedroom with frustration, some individuals may not have as strong an association between their bed and sleep-related frustration. In such cases, they may benefit from in-bed relaxation strategies that help them transition into sleep without leaving the bed.

- Janisha, a 40-year-old postal worker, has always viewed her bedroom as a place of relaxation. Even during bouts of insomnia, she doesn't associate her bed with frustration. She practices deep breathing exercises and progressive muscle relaxation techniques in bed, creating a sense of serenity that helps her transition into sleep.

Client Preferences: Ultimately, the effectiveness of insomnia management strategies should consider the preferences and comfort levels of the individual. Some clients may find it more distressing to get out of bed than to stay in bed and practice relaxation. It's crucial to tailor the approach to what works best for each client.

- David, a 50-year-old IT professional, prefers to stay in bed when he can't sleep as leaving the bed heightens his restlessness and anxiety. Instead, he reads a book under a dim bedside lamp, which brings him comfort and often leads to drowsiness, allowing him to fall asleep according to his preference.

Our exploration of sleep health in modern society underscores the need for a personalized, flexible approach. By embracing the individuality of each client's sleep journey and acknowledging these complexities, we foster a more inclusive and effective client education process. The ultimate measure of success in this journey is not just the quantity of sleep but the quality of restfulness, answering the soulful question, "Do I feel rested?" This approach aligns with our philosophy of respecting each client's unique sleep experience, guiding them towards a state of rest that is both satisfying and rejuvenating.

Many clients are already well-acquainted with the plethora of products and remedies marketed towards insomnia sufferers. Rather than regurgitating a list of potential solutions, we should harness the power of profound conversation, blending our clinical knowledge with genuine empathy and active listening. It's in this space of understanding and connection that we'll find the most effective, tailored approach for our client.

References

Akin-Little, A., & Little, S. G. (2019). Effect of extrinsic reinforcement on "intrinsic" motivation: Separating fact from fiction. In S. G. Little & A. Akin-Little (Eds.), Behavioral interventions in schools: Evidence-based positive strategies., 2nd ed. (pp. 113–132). American Psychological Association. https://doi.org/10.1037/0000126-007

Baillargeon, L., Landreville, P., Verreault, R., Beauchemin, J. P., Gregoire, J. P., & Morin, C. M. (2003). Discontinuation of benzodiazepines among older insomniac adults treated with cognitive-behavioural therapy combined with gradual tapering: A randomized trial. Canadian Medical Association Journal, 169, 1015–1020.

Bates, J. A. (1979). Extrinsic reward and intrinsic motivation: A review with implications for the classroom. Review of Educational Research, 49, 557–576. http://dx.doi.org/10.3102/00346543049004557

Belleville, G., & Morin, C. M. (2008). Hypnotic discontinuation in chronic insomnia: Impact of psychological distress, readiness to change, and self-efficacy. Health Psychology, 27, 239–248.

Buysse, Daniel J. Sleep Health: Can We Define It? Does It Matter?, *Sleep*, Volume 37, Issue 1, January 2014, Pages 9–17, https://doi.org/10.5665/sleep.3298

Cahn, S. C., Langenbucher, J. W., Friedman, M. A., Reavey, P., Falco, T., & Pallay, R. M. (2005). Predictors of interest in psychological treatment for insomnia among older primary care patients with disturbed sleep. Behavioral Sleep Medicine, 3(2), 87–98. https://doi.org/10.1207/s15402010bsm0302_3

Castelnovo, A., Ferri, R., Punjabi, N. M., Castronovo, V., Garbazza, C., Zucconi, M., Ferini-Strambi, L., & Manconi, M. (2019). The paradox of paradoxical insomnia: A theoretical review towards a unifying evidence-based definition. *Sleep Medicine Reviews*, *44*, 70–82. https://doi.org/10.1016/j.smrv.2018.12.007

Center for Self-Determination Theory. (2023). Intrinsic Motivation Inventory (IMI). Center for Self-Determination Theory. https://www.selfdeterminationtheory.org/IMI

Cerasoli, C. P., Nicklin, J. M., & Ford, M. T. (2014). Intrinsic motivation and extrinsic incentives jointly predict performance: A 40-year meta-analysis. Psychological Bulletin, 140, 980–1008. http://dx.doi.org/10.1037/a0035661

Deci, E. L., Koestner, R., & Ryan, R. M. (1999a). A meta-analytic review of experiments examining the effects of extrinsic rewards on intrinsic motivation. Psychological Bulletin, 125, 627–668. http://dx.doi.org/10.1037/0033-2909.125.6.627

Delaney, M. L., & Royal, M. A. (2017). Breaking engagement apart: The role of intrinsic and extrinsic motivation in engagement strategies. Industrial and Organizational Psychology: Perspectives on Science and Practice, 10, 127–140. http://dx.doi.org/10.1017/iop.2017.2

Disorders: A Comprehensive Primer of Behavioral Sleep Medicine Treatment Protocols. 1st ed. Cambridge, MA: Academic Press; 2011:143–149.

Dyrberg, H., Juel, A., & Kragh, M. (2021). Experience of Treatment and Adherence to Cognitive Behavioral Therapy for Insomnia for Patients with Depression: An Interview Study. Behavioral Sleep Medicine, 19(4), 481–491. https://doi.org/10.1080/15402002.2020.1788033

Edinger JD, Buysse DJ, Deriy L, Germain A, Lewin DS, Ong JC, Morgenthaler TI. Quality measures for the care of patients with insomnia. J Clin Sleep Med. 2015;11(3):311–334

Finlayson, J. G. (2013). The Persistence of Normative Questions in Habermas's Theory of Communicative Action. Constellations: An International Journal of Critical & Democratic Theory, 20(4), 518–532. https://doi.org/10.1111/1467-8675.12058

Germain A, Buysse DJ. Brief behavioral treatment of insomnia. In: Perlis M, Alioa M, Kuhn B, eds. Behavioral Treatments for Sleep

Grandner, Michael, Antonio Olivieri, Ajay Ahuja, Alexander Büsser, Moritz Freidank, & William V. McCall. (2023). The burden of untreated insomnia disorder in a sample of 1 million adults: a cohort study. *BMC Public Health*, *23*(1), 1–14. https://doi.org/10.1186/s12889-023-16329-9

Heath, S. (2017, August 15). Top 4 Patient Motivation Techniques for Health Improvement. Patient Engagement HIT. Retrieved from https://www.patientengagementhit.com

Lichstein, K. L., Nau, S. D., Wilson, N. M., et al. (2013). Psychological treatment of hypnotic-dependent insomnia in a primarily older adult sample. Behaviour Research and Therapy, 51, 787–796.

Linehan, M. M. (2015). DBT skills training manual (2nd ed.). New York, NY: Guilford Press.

Miller, W. R., & Moyers, T. B. (2017). Motivational interviewing and the clinical science of Carl Rogers. *Journal of Consulting and Clinical Psychology*, *85*(8), 757–766. https://doi.org/10.1037/ccp0000179

Miller, W. R., & Rose, G. S. (2015). Motivational interviewing and decisional balance: contrasting responses to client ambivalence. *Behavioural and Cognitive Psychotherapy*, *43*(2), 129–141. https://doi.org/10.1017/S1352465813000878

Morgenthaler, T., Kramer, M., Alessi, C., et al. (2006). American Academy of Sleep Medicine. Practice parameters for the psychological and behavioral treatment of insomnia: An update. Sleep, 29, 1415–1419.

Morin, C. M., Bastien, C., Guay, B., Radouco-Thomas, M., Leblanc, J., & Vallières, A. (2004). Randomized clinical trial of supervised tapering and cognitive behavior therapy to facilitate benzodiazepine discontinuation in older adults with chronic insomnia. American Journal of Psychiatry, 161, 332–342.

Morin, C. M., Bei, B., Bjorvatn, B., Poyares, D., Spiegelhalder, K., & Wing, Y. K. (2023). World sleep society international sleep medicine guidelines position statement endorsement of "behavioral and psychological treatments for chronic insomnia disorder in adults: An American Academy of sleep medicine clinical practice guidelines." *Sleep Medicine*, *109*, 164–169. https://doi.org/10.1016/j.sleep.2023.07.001

Morin, C. M., Bootzin, R. R., Buysse, D. J., Edinger, J. D., Espie, C. A., & Lichstein, K. L. (2006). Psychological and behavioral treatment of insomnia: Update of the recent evidence (1998–2004). Sleep, 29, 1398–1414.

Norcross, J. C. (2013). *Self-help that works: evidence-based resources for the public and the professional* (Fourth edition.). Oxford University Press.

Ntoumanis, N., Ng, J. Y. Y., Prestwich, A., Quested, E., Hancox, J. E., Thøgersen-Ntoumani, C., Deci, E. L., Ryan, R. M., Lonsdale, C., & Williams, G. C. (2021). A meta-analysis of self-determination theory-informed intervention studies in the health domain: effects on motivation, health behavior, physical, and psychological health. Health Psychology Review, 15(2), 214–244. https://doi.org/10.1080/17437199.2020.1718529

O'Connor, K. P., Marchand, A., Belanger, L., et al. (2004). Psychological distress and adaptational problems associated with benzodiazepine withdrawal and outcome: A replication. Addictive Behaviors, 29, 583–593.

Okajima, I., Nakamura, M., Nishida, S., et al. (2013). Cognitive behavioural therapy with behavioural analysis for pharmacological treatment-resistant chronic insomnia. Psychiatry Research, 210, 515–521.

Poyer, J. (2023, April 1). Insomnia Doc's Guide to Restful Sleep: Remedies for Insomnia and Good Sleep Health. *Library Journal, 148*(4), 58.

Prochaska, J. O., DiClemente, C. C., Lipkus, I. M., McBride, C. M., Bloom, P. N., Pollak, K. I., Schwartz-Bloom, R. D., & Tilson, E. (2004). Stages of Change Questionnaire. *Health Psychology, 23*, 397–406.

Ren, J., & Wang, N. (2018). A Survey of Students' Motivation in College English Learning under Production-Oriented Approach in NCEPU. English Language Teaching, 11(12), 199–204.

Sateia MJ, Buysse DJ, Krystal AD, Neubauer DN, Heald JL. Clinical practice guideline for the pharmacologic treatment of chronic insomnia in adults: American Academy of Sleep Medicine clinical practice guideline. J Clin Sleep Med. 2017;13(2):307–349.

Schutte-Rodin S, Broch L, Buysse D, Dorsey C, Sateia M. Clinical guideline for the evaluation and management of chronic insomnia in adults. J Clin Sleep Med. 2008;4(5):487–504. 13.

Shulman, L. (1986). Those who understand: Knowledge growth in teaching. Educational Researcher, 15(2), 4–14.

Shulman, L. S. (2000). Teacher development: Roles of domain expertise and pedagogical knowledge. Journal of Applied Developmental Psychology, 21(1), 129–135.

Sommers-Flanagan, J., & Sommers-Flanagan, R. (2015). *Clinical interviewing*. John Wiley & Sons, Incorporated.

Troxel WM, Germain A, Buysse DJ. Clinical management of insomnia with brief behavioral treatment (BBTI). Behav Sleep Med. 2012;10(4):266–279.

Vidusha, Paul K., Thilagar, S., Lakshmanan, D. K., Ravichandran, G., & Arunachalam, A. (2022). Advancement in the contemporary clinical diagnosis and treatment strategies of insomnia disorder. *Sleep Medicine*, *91*, 124–140. https://doi.org/10.1016/j.sleep.2022.02.018

Walseth, L. T., Abildsnes, E., & Schei, E. (2011). Patients' experiences with lifestyle counselling in general practice: A qualitative study. Scandinavian Journal of Primary Health Care, 29(2), 99–103. https://doi.org/10.3109/02813432.2011.553995

Whiteman, Rodney S. (2015). Explicating metatheory for mixed methods research in educational leadership : An application of Habermas's Theory of Communicative Action. International Journal of Educational Management, 29(7), 888–903. https://doi.org/10.1108/IJEM-06-2015-0077

Yang, C.-M., Tseng, C.-H., Lai, Y.-S., & Hsu, S.-C. (2008). Behavioral therapies for insomnia: The importance of variability among older adults. Aging & Mental Health, 12(1), 51–61.

About the Author

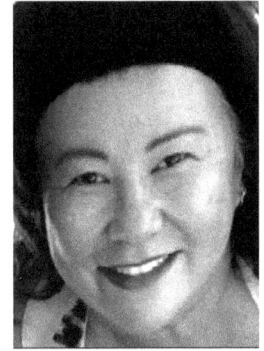Linda Rosenbery is a seasoned mental health counselor and the Managing Director of a sleep medicine practice and CPAP Durable Medical Equipment company in the Chicago area. With a career spanning multiple roles, her current work can be characterized by a quiet passion to integrate clinical expertise with empathetic dialogue in the treatment of insomnia. She is deeply committed to filling the service gap in specialized insomnia therapy. Linda holds profound respect for, and is guided by, leading institutions in sleep medicine, including the American Academy of Sleep Medicine, the National Sleep Foundation, and the sleep research programs at Cleveland Clinic, Stanford, and the University of Pittsburgh.

www.ingramcontent.com/pod-product-compliance
Lightning Source LLC
LaVergne TN
LVHW070526070526
838199LV00073B/6713